OLDER AMERICANS,
VITAL COMMUNITIES

OLDER AMERICANS, VITAL COMMUNITIES

A Bold Vision for Societal Aging

W. ANDREW ACHENBAUM

THE JOHNS HOPKINS UNIVERSITY PRESS
BALTIMORE

© 2005 The Johns Hopkins University Press
All rights reserved. Published 2005
Printed in the United States of America on acid-free paper
9 8 7 6 5 4 3 2 1

The Johns Hopkins University Press
2715 North Charles Street
Baltimore, Maryland 21218-4363
www.press.jhu.edu

Library of Congress Cataloging-in-Publication Data
Achenbaum, W. Andrew.
    Older Americans, vital communities : a bold vision for societal aging /
W. Andrew Achenbaum.
        p.   cm.
    Includes bibliographical references and index.
    ISBN 0-8018-8237-0 (hardcover : alk. paper)
    1. Older people—United States—Social conditions—21st century. 2. Longevity—Social
aspects—United States. 3. Social change—United States. 4. Self-actualization (Psychology) in
old age—United States. 5. Older people—Government policy—United States. 6. Social
prediction—United States—21st century. I. Title.
    HQ1064.U5A6254 2005
    305.26′0973—dc22   2005005203

A catalog record for this book is available from the British Library.

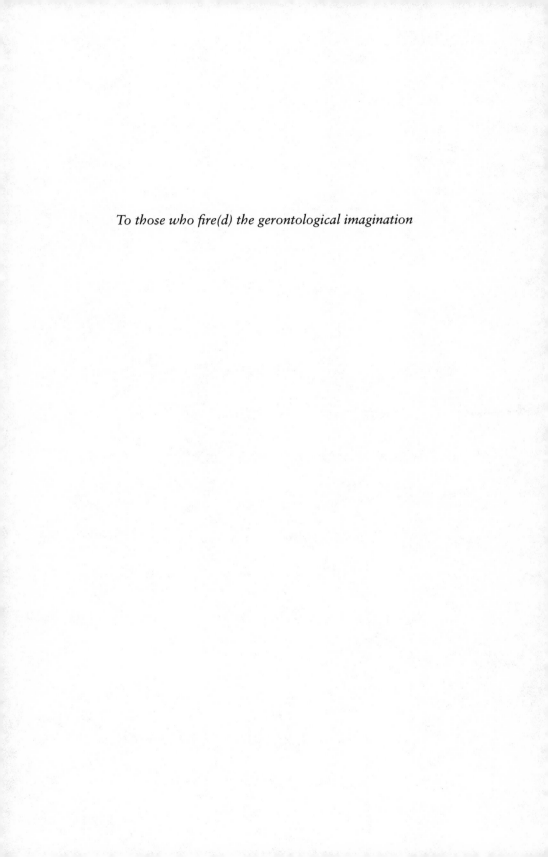

To those who fire(d) the gerontological imagination

CONTENTS

ACKNOWLEDGMENTS

I first started thinking about the themes of this book when I served in the mid-1980s on The Aging Society Project sponsored by the Carnegie Corporation of New York. I owe a special debt of gratitude to Alan Pifer and the late Lydia Bronte for inviting me to participate. *Older Americans, Vital Communities* is my way of extending the themes and arguments they incubated.

An earlier version of chapter 4 was presented to colleagues at the Institute for Medical Humanities, University of Texas Medical Branch, Galveston.

Wendy Harris edited my first book, *Old Age in the New Land*. Over the past twenty-five years, she has remained a sounding board with an eye for details sharper than ever. William Kelly assisted me with last-minute editing, a service he has rendered since we were in college. I also wish to thank the copyeditor, Elizabeth Yoder, for getting the book ready for print, and the production editor, Andre Barnett.

I have dedicated this study to gerontology's pioneers. Over the years, many have become intellectual sojourners, and a few are dear friends. Although none should be held accountable for the contents of this book, I thank the following for firing my imagination: Dick Adelman, Toni Antonucci, Bob Applebaum, Bob Atchley, Jeanne Bader, Bob Ball, Scott Bass, Vern Bengtson, Bob Binstock, Jim and Betty Birren, Lenore Epstein Bixby, Andrew Blaikie, Fred Bookstein, Dana Bradley, Tom Brown, Bob

Butler, Bing Chen, Li-Mei Chen, Wilbur Cohen, Tom Cole, Jack Cornman, Neal Cutler, Stephen Cutler, Gerson David, Rose Dobrof, Wilma Donahue, Libby Douvan, David Ekherdt, Glen Elder, Joan and Erik Erikson, Carroll Estes, Stephanie Fallingcreek, Tuck Finch, Arthur Flemming, Lawrence Frank, Joe Freeman, Brant Fries, Linda George, Rose Gibson, Margaret Gullette, David Gutmann, Carole Haber, Jeff Halter, Gunhild Hagestad, Leonard Hayflick, Joe Hendricks, Regula Herzog, James Jackson, Malcolm Johnson, Paul Johnson, Rosalie Kane, Bob Kastenbaum, Stephen Katz, Gary Kenyon, Eric Kingson, Maggie Kuhn, Jim Kvale, Frieder Lang, Peter Laslett, Powell Lawton, Jeff Levin, Helen Lopata, George Maddox, Ron Manheimer, Koko Markides, Victor Marshall, Rich Miller, Rick Moody, Bob Morris, Malcolm Morrison, Barbara Myerhoff, Bob Myers, John Myles, Bernice Neugarten, Mary O'Brien, Bill Oriol, Barbara Payne, Marion Perlmutter, Henry Pratt, Jill Quadagno, Joe Quinn, Klaus Riegel, Matilda and Jack Riley, Dorrie Rosenblatt, Carolyn Rosenthal, Irving Rosow, Jack Rother, Jack Rowe, Carol Ryff, Andrea Sankar, Jim Schulz, Carol Schutz, Millie Seltzer, Ethel Shanas, Nathan Shock, Herb Shore, Mickey Smyer, Jay Sokolovsky, Peter Stearns, Robyn Stone, Bernie Strehler, Gordon Strieb, Jim Sykes, Sheldon Tobin, Fernando Torres-Gil, Lillian Troll, David Van Tassel, Lois Verbrugge, Tony Warnes, Bill Wasch, Larry Weiss, Fox Wetle, Nancy Whitelaw, and Carter Williams.

Finally, I thank my family, friends, and colleagues for their loving support during good times and bad.

INTRODUCTION
A New Demographic Revolution
Demands Novel Structural Responses

The simple fact that more and more of us are living longer and longer is bringing profound changes to our personal identities. Meanwhile, the broader social fabric is aging. This often causes lags and gaps in institutional capabilities and in their capacities to meet human needs. Structures sometimes thwart men and women who want to take full advantage of the extra years before them.

This volume surveys how the extension of the human life course will affect virtually all elements of our nation's mosaic. Population aging has already transformed institutions and altered relationships. Less dramatic than terrorism, less visible than environmental decay, the consequences of extra years have yet to receive sustained attention. Few of us look much beyond the present moment to envision our future selves in different economic, social, spiritual, political, familial, and global arrangements. This book recounts what has and has not been done so far to accommodate various segments of our society's diverse population as they mature. It pays special attention to the so-called baby boomers, who are positioned by historical circumstances to modify and create organizational structures to promote productive, vital growth for the common good. And it challenges today's younger generations to think more boldly about the long lives that lie before them.

As such, the argument of this book runs against many habits of thought. Most of the college students I know operate on a very short timeline. They make elaborate plans for the upcoming weekend but fail to wonder about what may be in store for them past the age of thirty. Even my brightest undergraduates look surprised when I ask them if they have given any thought to where they want to be, much less what they hope to be doing, when they reach their parents' age. In my thirty years of teaching, no one has expressed interest in mapping a path that extends another six decades, bringing them into the later years that will likely be theirs.

Reading this book can help students imagine their futures in fresh ways. They will no doubt continue to mark time mainly in terms of days and months, but this book should sensitize them to the contingent nature of life experiences. Students will discover that the power to create new structures and human bonds extends into advanced years. They will be led to think anew about the past as prologue. In *Democracy in America,* Alexis de Tocqueville might well have been describing my students when he wrote: "Those who went before are soon forgotten; of those who will come after, no one has any idea" (194).

To be fair, undergraduates are not the only ones who have trouble grasping the shape of time, and this book speaks to their elders as well. Few adults make provisions for disruptions in their routines. Nor, given their commitments to family and colleagues, are many in the prime of their lives willing to risk taking advantage of new opportunities. "Future shock," according to Alvin Toffler (1970) is particularly acute among the baby boom generation. My cohort, born in an era of affluence, seemed destined to transform American society by dint of our numbers and energy. We received the best our parents could afford. The educational system expanded as we moved from kindergarten through graduate school. Our music, our social mores, and our political protests redefined American culture in the 1960s. In middle age, though, we are rarely perceived as agents of cultural change. Some of us dropped out; others sold out. Most of us struggle to get by. Few have found havens as comfortable as we desired—or conditions as boring as we feared. Midlife for many men and women born between 1946 and 1964 affords moments for introspection and redirection.

The central premise offered here is that a historical perspective is essential for all of us, young and old, to develop a fuller perspective on our lengthening life spans. Experience teaches a lot. Still, it is difficult to graft a nebulous future onto a historical timeline. "Nothing ever becomes real till it is experienced," John Keats wrote in a letter in 1818 (quoted in Forman, 1952: 316). Temporal guideposts point the way while we are exploring uncharted territories.

As a historian, I know that some facets of the human condition are universal. Mortals are born to die. In between, we work, play, eat, sleep, love, fight, adapt to our environment, and interact with other living creatures. We feel emotions such as hope, anger, inspiration, jealousy, euphoria, and depression. Fears, anxieties, and moments of bliss are part of the human experience too. The context in which we live out our days alters with time. Most such historical changes, I have learned, unfold slowly. Cumulatively, they necessitate only minor modifications in prevailing ideas, activities, and relationships. Sometimes the temporal accretions prompt a reconsideration of traditional institutions and mores; at other times they modify conventional ways of seeing and doing things. Some historical trends, especially in the arts and commerce, occur in cycles. And finally, some events (such as 9/11) are truly revolutionary in scope: they represent a "deep change . . . [a] change in the *rate* of change—an alteration which is at once discontinuous in its nature and transforming in its effect" (Fischer, 1977: 100).

Given the multifaceted influences of time on the intricate, fragile human enterprise, historical changes are usually asynchronous (Kubler, 1962). Cultural and structural lags are pandemic in world history and throughout our nation's experience. Many critical divisions and disjunctures in U.S. history, so familiar as to require merely brief note, occurred in divergent ways and at different rates. Novel technologies, new modes of transportation, and economic innovations, among other things, caused disparities among Americans. Some of the polarities were experienced along geographic lines—east/west, north/south, urban/rural. In distinctive ways, diverse institutions—ranging from slavery; to access to schools and colleges, corporations, reform movements; to political parties and government agencies—benefited some groups and disadvantaged others. To this must be added ways that demographic diversity—black and white, male and female, native born and foreign born, members of religious sects and denominations, rich and poor—affected chances for upward mobility.

I have chosen to focus on the history of "age" in America, which is full of examples in which institutional structures did not support prevailing assumptions about specific stages of the life course. For instance, parents and the citizenry have always invested hope and resources in children and youth, making education a priority. Public schools were charged with teaching skills needed in the marketplace, promoting patriotism, and (later on) socializing children for adulthood (Hall, 1904; Fass, 1978). But results were uneven for most of our history. African Americans, when not denied access to learning, were consigned to inferior, segregated educational facilities. Gender bias limited females' curricular options and career tracks. Many immigrants wanted their offspring to supplement the family economy rather than become literate or Americanized. Roman Catholics built parochial schools to ensure that their youth received proper religious instruction. Meanwhile, state and federal lawmakers, notably in the periods of the Progressive era, the Depression, and the Great Society, created institutions to provide medical care and social services for the young. How ironic, then, that today children under 18 constitute the highest proportion of the nation's poor. The daughters and sons of minorities are most at risk to be left behind, victims of neglect, abuse, and inadequate health care (Kett, 1977; Pleck, 1991).

Segments of the middle-aged population faced a different set of institutional barriers. Workers were denied jobs on the basis of race and ethnicity, and sometimes religion. Disabled persons were marginalized. Women's right to work outside of the home was limited, and they were denied the right to vote until 1920. Despite such obstacles and prejudice, female reformers from all backgrounds played a crucial role in creating social welfare facilities and charities. Women artists and writers helped to craft a distinctive American idiom.

"Old age is not interesting until one gets there," May Sarton observed in *As We Are Now*. It is "a foreign country with an unknown language to the young and even to the middle-aged" (1973: 23). The discontinuities of late life have become truly apparent in the twentieth century. There are more than twice as many Americans over 65 today as in 1960. Gender differences in morbidity and mortality, economic dependency, and social support make the "modern" history of old age a prominent component of women's studies. Old-age dependency was once left to individuals, families, and the local community to handle. (Veterans' benefits, which accounted for most of the funds allocated to elderly citizens before 1929, were not considered old-age programs.) Now, however, Social Security and elder care are major foci of federal policymakers, spurred by a gray lobby keen to increase age-based entitlements (Haber, 1983; Haber and Grattan, 1994; Cole, 1992).

So far, remarkably little consideration has been paid to societal aging, although the median age of the population has doubled since 1790. In the late eighteenth century, people on both sides of the Atlantic followed a debate sparked by Thomas Robert Malthus, William Godwin, and Antoine-Nicolas de Condorcet over the possibility and desirability of prolonging human life. Considering longevity an accurate gauge of the environmental, social, and political health of a polity, Americans gathered bills of mortality to "prove" that living in the New World contributed to long life and good government (Achenbaum, 1978a: 12–13). In the late nineteenth century, the presumptive benefits of population aging were displaced by negative opinions first uttered in Europe: commentators ascribed the defeat of French forces in the Franco-Prussian War (1870) to the country's low birth rate.

The contemporary study of population aging in the United States commenced in 1929 when President Herbert Hoover invited a distinguished group of academics and public officials to survey *Recent Social Trends* (President's Research Committee, 1933). Elaborating themes in their 1930 article in the *American Mercury*, "A Nation of Elders in the Making," Warren S. Thompson and P. K. Whelpton reported that "age changes are likely to produce significant consequences in our schools, in our business, in our politics and in our social structure. . . . Such developments in turn may influence the outlook and taste of the whole population" (57, 36).

While New Dealers rarely consulted Hoover's *Recent Social Trends,* they did have population aging in mind as they designed the foundations of the nation's welfare state. Visions of an age-integrated society determined features of the 1935 Social Security Act. Old-age assistance and insurance, Congress hoped, would reduce the long-term costs to the young in providing funds for elders. Public health services were intended to improve the well-being of mothers and children in rural America, reducing risks later in life. The 1939 Social Security amendments, moreover, presumed that "the protection of the aged must not be at the expense of adequate protection of dependent children, the sick, the disabled or the unemployed" (Brown, 1977: 18).

A transgenerational approach to Social Security through interconnected institutional domains did not, unfortunately, take root. Instead,

Social Security administrators guarded their turf and cultivated allies to protect their programs. Categorical initiatives became compartmentalized, thwarting cooperative partnerships within the system and with other federal agencies (Achenbaum, 1986). Policymakers after World War II engaged in "the politics of incrementalism," expanding the scope of existing provisions under their aegis. Administrators who put their agencies' needs first rarely connected with other related age-specific programs in the public or private sector.

Population aging, a few scholars warned after World War II, would affect the course of cold war politics. Americans would "need to learn about the consequences of the aging of nations," opined University of Chicago's Philip Hauser: "If youth means vigor and age debility, the Western and free nations may be handicapped. . . . But youth has not always triumphed over age, and age has many virtues not possessed by youth" (Hauser and Vargas, 1960: 52). Fifteen years later, two of Hauser's colleagues directed a National Science Foundation project probing *Social Policy, Social Ethics, and the Aging Society* (Neugarten and Havighurst, 1976). By the early 1980s, reports on the impact of population aging were issued by President Jimmy Carter, the U.S. Senate Special Committee on Aging, and several gerontology centers. Rarely defining what they meant by "societal aging," experts tended to focus on older Americans while downplaying their relationships with the young and middle-aged populations.

Indeed, U.S. attempts to probe the consequences of societal aging seem modest compared to efforts elsewhere. In 1960 Japanese leaders began to track the impact of increases in life expectancy at birth and in middle age after World War II because the population was experiencing enormous gains in longevity over the life course. The Japanese Economic Council convened a group of 128 experts in the 1980s to prepare their country "for an age of internationalization, the aging society and maturity" (Economic Council, 1983: 139; Ibe, 2000). Scholars and politicians in Australia and New Zealand also generated ideas about societal aging. Concerns in Europe over sustaining welfare programs amid fiscal restraint spurred heated discussions about population aging and economic dependency (P. Johnson, 1987).

During the past two decades, American scholars have joined peers overseas to assess the effect of population aging on advanced industrial societies. Robert N. Butler, M.D., the first director of the National Institute on Aging and Pulitzer Prize–winning author of *Why Survive?* (1975), launched an International Longevity Center with Japanese colleagues. The Carnegie Corporation underwrote major studies of population aging in both the United States and the United Kingdom. Alan Pifer and Lydia Bronte brought together a group of scholars, critics, and leaders in the corporate and philanthropic sectors to design a special edition of *Daedalus* (1986a), which was then published as *Our Aging Society* (1986b). Like their predecessors, the authors focused on certain population groups, on specific social policies, and on particular sectors of the economy. They designated Americans between the ages of 50 and 75, those in the so-called third quarter of life, as catalysts of change. But few contributors sufficiently differentiated between individual development and societal aging.

Nations and institutions do not "age" like ordinary human beings. Nation states do not have "natural" life spans. Increasing fertility rates rejuvenate nation states, whereas individuals only grow older. Nor do mature societies inevitably stagnate and die after a prescribed number of decades. Similarly, lawmakers prefer to make incremental changes in social legislation, earmarking a percentage of funds to older persons and distributing other resources to other groups. They rarely talk about continuities across the life course. Nor do they often bring bureaucrats, experts, and advocates from one domain (say, the environment) together with those advocating child welfare. Finally, lawmakers, like their constituencies, tend to focus on "crises." Population aging has been evolving unobtrusively for so long that other domestic and international matters will take precedence until the demographic "time bomb" (if that is what it is) has to be defused.

Several contributors to *Our Aging Society* continued to address population aging after the Carnegie project ended. Bernice Neugarten, who coined the term *societal aging,* excoriated social policies based on age, not need. Fernando Torres-Gil, who served as the nation's first assistant secretary for aging in the Clinton administration, forged institutional coalitions between disabled persons and the nation's elders. To combat age-segregated policy-making, Torres-Gil urged older Americans to support public funding for schools, to fight the war on drugs, and to stay active (1992: 89–90). Matilda White Riley and her husband, John W.

Riley, started their Program on Age and Structural Change through the National Institute on Aging to investigate how the longevity revolution would diversify opportunities along the life course:

> The tendency for structural changes to lag behind changes in people's lives has become a serious problem in our lives. . . . We have entered a historical period in which men and women live, on average, almost 20 years beyond the usual retirement age . . . an extended period of older age that is essentially without formal structure, an entry into the time of the "roleless role." The contrast between these life stages is increasingly visible and increasingly conflict prone, especially as the economic entitlements of older people are often seen as economic burdens of the young and middle-aged. . . . We have complex problems to solve in bringing our opportunity structures . . . into greater congruence with what medical and the technological advances have done for the way we grow up and grow old. (Riley, Kahn, and Foner, 1994: vii–viii)

One source of the structural lag, the Rileys and their associates argued, was the prevalence of "three boxes of life"—education for the young, work and family for the middle-aged, and retirement and leisure for the old—which did not foster the potential for increased productivity through a more flexible, imaginative use of human resources.

Not all commentators and public officials were as sanguine as the Rileys about the positive impact of population aging on U.S. society. As the baby boomers entered middle age, columnists such as Philip Longman warned that they would "become the first cohort of senior citizens unable to draw on the economic output and financial support of a much larger number of younger Americans" (1987: 3). The resources needed to provide retirement benefits and healthcare support for increasing numbers of senior citizens alarmed conservatives in an era of fiscal restraint. Longman succeeded in raising a critical policy question: Did the potentially deleterious consequences of population aging justify a reduction in old-age entitlements?

Longman's jeremiad complemented a neoconservative vision of the political economy then dominating Washington. In the wake of the 1983 crisis over Social Security financing, two congressional representatives founded Americans for Generational Equity (AGE) as a "lobby for the future." AGE claimed that the "downward mobility of the baby boomers has compounded with a vengeance on their children" (Van Tassel and

Meyer, 1992: 39). After questionable financial dealings crippled AGE, Peter Peterson (a former secretary of commerce) and several U.S. senators created the Concord Coalition in 1992. Supported by more than 200,000 members, the coalition called "for an end to federal budget deficits, for equitable Social Security and Medicare reform, for stronger long-term economic growth, and for a higher standard of living for future generations of Americans." A failure of nerve, Peterson repeatedly claimed in the media, would make the United States "a nation in decline—with a faltering economy, reduced international influence, and lowered expectations for all" (Peterson and Howe, 1988: 4).

Concern for the rights and interests of unborn generations is not new. "Can one generation bind another, and all others, in succession forever?" asked Thomas Jefferson rhetorically in 1824. "A generation may bind itself as long as its majority continues in life; when that has disappeared, another majority is in place, holds all the rights and powers their predecessors once held, and may change their laws and institutions to suit themselves" (Koch and Peden, 1944: 714). Updating Jefferson's query, David M. Walker, comptroller of the United States under Presidents Bill Clinton and George W. Bush, contended that institutional changes in the workplace were necessary to prevent the negative consequences associated with the global implications of population aging (Walker, 2002, 2003). A failure to confront the dangers inherent in population aging, warned George Will (2002), would have dire consequences: "Aging populations, declining birthrates, and intolerance of invigorating immigration make for long-term economic anemia."

There was a middle ground. Some scholars contended that population aging was not catastrophic, the source of all imminent woes. "Fears of future crises have as much to do with current institutional arrangements as with the characteristics of old people," declared William Jackson. "If the social institutions surrounding old age could be made more diversified and less restrictive, so as to match the diversity of the elderly population, then there would be little reason to worry about population ageing" (1998: 206; see also Mullan, 2000; Posner, 1995). Agreeing that *Demography Is Not Destiny*, the National Academy on an Aging Society (1999: 19) argued that the critical policy issue was sustaining productivity. Future financing of federal old-age entitlements *would* be difficult if the United States experienced little or no economic growth. Institutions, however, could be adapted to promote growth.

This volume joins the debate over societal aging by examining the interplay between aging cohorts and institutional contexts from a historical perspective. It acknowledges that a variety of conflicting dreams and forecasts about the future condition does not preclude a patient, steady gaze on an agenda that puts a premium on advancing individual capacities while promoting social justice (Kateb, 1963). We can learn from experience if we think of population aging in terms of past trends, present circumstances, and future possibilities. Despite our penchant for operating on short timelines, we need to take a long view. All age groups, not just one cohort, must embark on *terra incognita*. If we wait much longer to act, it will be harder to adapt our basic institutions to accommodate a future that we desire.

In contemplating life's uncertain journey, we must exercise our imagination. "The great instrument of moral good is imagination," the poet Percy Bysshe Shelley declared. "We have more moral, political, and historical wisdom than we know how to reduce into practice; we have more scientific and economic knowledge than can be accommodated to the just distribution of the produce which it multiplies" (quoted in Clark, ed., 1954: 283, 293). To adapt to population aging, we must envision how basic societal institutions can generate new structural incentives, enabling people to contribute throughout their lives.

The discussion begins in chapter 1 with an overview of the new faces of aging. Acknowledging the importance of extra years of life expectancy, it pays particular attention to women's issues as well as to ethnic and racial diversity. Chapter 2 deals with "productive aging," suggesting ways to make trade-offs between work and leisure. This discussion leads to chapter 3 on "vital aging," which emphasizes the need for wise learning at all stages of life. Chapter 4 emphasizes that fighting ageism and changing the way we train physicians would advance healthful aging. Chapter 5 focuses on the recent growth of "spiritual aging" in theory and practice. Chapter 6 considers the ties that bind age groups together; it starts with a discussion of global aging and ends with the family, a little commonwealth. The epilogue affirms the creativity of older people to revivify culture if given the opportunity and support. Highlighting the symbiotic relationship between individual choices and institutional responsibilities, it ends by challenging the baby boomers to be trailblazers as members of their particular networks and as citizens of the world.

The New Faces of Individual Aging } 1

By any measure, the U.S. population has been aging since the founding of the republic. The median age of the population, according to the 1790 Federal Census, was 16. Half the population was under the age of 20 on the eve of the Civil War. As late as 1950, only half the U.S. population was over 30. Population aging has accelerated during the past half-century. The median age rose to 34 by 1994. In that year there were as many people over 60 as there were children under 14. Half of all Americans will be over 39 by 2030, demographers project (Hobbs and Damon, 1996: v, 1-1). The number of men and women over 65 has increased elevenfold since 1900, far outstripping the threefold growth among those under 65. The number of centenarians has more than doubled in the United States since 1980.

As a result of population aging, America's age structure has changed its shape. In 1905 the distribution resembled a triangle, wide at the bottom (because of the large number of births) and narrow at the top (because death thinned the ranks of middle-aged and older adults). By 2050, according to best estimates, the pyramid will look more like a rectangle (U.S. Bureau of Census, 1960; Hobbs and Damon: 2-5, 2-7). Three factors will cause this transformation. First, continually declining fertility rates will increase the relative size of the older population. Second, advances in public health, pharmacology, and medical interventions should reduce the numbers of people who die in adulthood, postponing death until advanced years. And third, heavy immigration rates tended to rejuvenate the U.S. age structure in the past because younger people are more likely than elderly ones to move from abroad to this country. Barring a greater influx of foreign-born persons than anticipated, immigration will not greatly affect the shape of the nation's population structure.

The concatenation of declining fertility and mortality rates and minimal migration that accounts for U.S. population aging does not exist everywhere in the world. In recent decades there has been a significant growth south of the equator in the *absolute* numbers of men and women living past the age of 60. The *relative* growth in the proportion of older people in South America, Africa, and the subcontinent, however, has been dampened by the persistence of high fertility rates. Unlike their neighbors to the north, policymakers in developing countries have had to address simultaneously the different needs of two vulnerable subsets of their population, the very young and the very old.

Besides cross-national differences in population aging, it is worth noting that experts disagree about the future size of older cohorts in developed nations such as the United States. Some scientists theorize that genetic manipulation might someday extend the human life span indefinitely. Much controversy surrounds prospects of using drugs or hormones as interventions to reverse the processes of aging. Anti-aging medicine, as a way to enlarge and improve human life beyond present limits, has a long, although not auspicious, history (J. Smith, 2004). Eos, the Greek goddess of dawn, asked Zeus to give the Trojan prince Tithonos immortality. Her wish was granted, but she forgot to ask that her lover also be given eternal youth. Tithonos eventually shriveled into a wizened grasshopper (Hornblower and Spawforth, 1996: 526). In *Gulliver's Travels,* Swift's protagonist is filled with "sublunary happiness" as he learns new things about the stars and comets from the *struldbrugs,* beings that lived forever in the kingdom of Luggnagg. In due course, however, Gulliver discerned that immortality guaranteed neither vigor nor zest for life. The creatures became melancholy after thirty. Females of the species aged in a more frightful manner than males. By eighty, the *struldbrugs* had lost their hair, teeth, and appetites. The citizens of Luggnagg considered them legally dead. No longer able to communicate after their second century of life, the *struldbrugs* were despised by all (Swift, 1726: 225–31). Despite the specter of obsolescent, debilitating senility, the search for eternal youth has continued to fascinate mythologists, alchemists, and even scientists in both the East and the West since ancient times (Gruman, 1966). Elie Metchnikoff, the Nobel laureate who was convinced that eating yogurt delayed his death, declared it axiomatic that "it is useful to prolong life" (1908: 135). Americans spend billions of dollars to look youthful as long as possible. Thus far, however, attempts to extend the human life span have been unsuccessful.

Scientists have, nonetheless, increased longevity in the animal kingdom. Since the 1930s, gerontologists have extended the life span of certain invertebrates and vertebrates, including mammals, by substantially reducing their food intake. Mice and rats with limited access to food become smaller and lose some of their neurological capacities, but they live 30–50 percent longer than those of their species that are permitted to eat as they wish. Recent tests on monkeys, our closest evolutionary companions, indicate that caloric restriction lowers blood pressure and reduces chronic illnesses as compared to normal diets. It is too early, however, to determine whether dietary limitations increase their life spans (President's Council on Bioethics, 2003).

I assume here that there is a finite limit to the human life span—unless a dramatic breakthrough should occur. At present no scientific evidence contradicts Genesis 6:3, which states that "their days shall be one hundred twenty years." Scientists discount sensational reports of men and women living far beyond that age in the Andean highlands or Georgian mountains. Vital statistics have in most instances disputed claims of Civil War veterans, slaves, and widows reported to have lived to be 130 or 140. Although 120 years may not be the literal limit (some cite 122 as an alternative), it is a good approximation. Biomedical researchers hypothesize that if all forms of cancer, cardiovascular diseases, and diabetes were eliminated, life expectancy at birth in the United States would increase by a dozen years. Such an impressive gain would still fall far short of what some consider the maximum human life span. So what has been the cumulative increase in the number of years people expect to live? Current and historical demographic statistics enable us to map where we have been, where we are, and where we are likely to head (Dunn, 1992: xiv; Olshansky and Carnes, 2001).

According to the best available evidence, the average life expectancy at birth in ancient Greece was 30; in ancient Rome, 35. Hunters probably died at around age 25 (Hornblower and Spawforth, 1996: 38; Den-

neen, 2000). Most babies in ancient times died at birth. That said, those
in the Classical era who survived infancy and childhood sometimes managed to live to old age. Sparta was ruled by men in their sixties; *senator*
is derived from the Latin word *senex*, 'old.' According to Chinese tradition, Lao Tzu, born with white hair and the face of an old man, lived
past 80 (Chevalier and Gheerbrant, 1996: 715). The Patriarchs surely
did not live as long as recorded in Hebrew Scripture, but the reference
in Psalm 90 to the decline that occurs after age 80 strikes a contemporary note of truth (D. N. Freedman, 1992: V, 10–12).

Fragmentary evidence indicates that there was little change in life
expectancy at birth throughout most of recorded history. Since the fourteenth century, if not before, our ancestors in both the West and the East
did not expect to live much longer than the ancients (Kertzer and Laslett,
1994: 68; Ottaway et al., 2002). Calculating life expectancy data at age
15 as a way to circumvent the high morbidity and mortality rates associated with infancy and childhood does not alter the general trend, not-
withstanding variations in life expectancy at birth by generation, occupation, class, and family history.

The Demographic Dimensions of America's "New Old"

Consistent with this centuries-old pattern, life expectancy at birth was
about 35 at the founding of the New Republic. It increased to 42 in the
United States by the mid-1800s. Average life expectancy at birth increased five more years by 1900. Fifty years later, it jumped dramatically
to 68. According to the latest census data, average life expectancy at
birth for males was 74.4 years and for females 79.8 (Centers for Disease
Control, 2003: Table 27). In addition, there have been modest but noteworthy gains (3–4 years) in life expectancy at 50 and at 65. Each successive cohort of elders has managed to keep death at bay a bit longer
with the help of medical advances, better living conditions and diets,
and more effective preventive health measures. That two-thirds of the
improvement in longevity occurred in the twentieth century attests to an
unprecedented demographic transition. The percentage of elders grows
as the aging of American society itself becomes more pronounced (Riley
and Riley, 1986: 55). It is no wonder that the new faces of aging have
transformed how we think about age.

"Sixty-five" is no longer *the* benchmark signaling the onset of late life.
Those who are now 65 generally are healthier, wealthier, and more active

4

than was true of previous elderly cohorts, as is borne out by comparing findings from the 1974 and 2000 surveys conducted by the National Council on the Aging. Fewer 65-year-olds reported themselves in poor health in 2000 (42%) than in 1974 (54%). Only a fifth in the latest sample claimed that loneliness was a problem, compared to more than the third who said, when questioned in 1974, that they were isolated. Surprisingly, more than 40 percent of those surveyed in 2000 considered themselves middle-aged (rather than elderly) at 65. Today's cohort of elders think that the problems associated with growing older are not likely to arise until they reach 75 (Cutler, Whitelaw, and Beattie, 2002: vii–viii).

Indeed, the incidence of poverty and disease is more apparent at advanced ages than it was in the past, as more and more Americans live to age 85 and beyond. The "old-old" cohort of elders (those over 85) is the fastest-growing part of the aged population. In 1900 only 4 percent of those over 65 were over 85; by the end of the century, one in ten was over 85. Some predict that men and women over 85 will constitute nearly a fifth of all senior citizens by 2050. Between 1960 and 1994, this group increased in number by 274 percent compared to the 100 percent increase among all those over 65 (Hobbs and Damon, 1996: 2-8, 2-9). As we shall see, there is a wider range of competencies, capacities, and assets among the old-old than younger persons typically perceive. Stereotypes abound. Just as Americans in the 1970s belittled the potential contributions of those over 65, they now caricature those over 85. Ageism prevents many people of all ages from seeing that potentials are as bountiful as are problems among the very old.

Gender differences within the elderly population became increasingly important during the twentieth century. The proportions of older men and women in the U.S. population were virtually identical (4%) in 1900. In 1970, however, 11.2 percent of all American females were over 65, compared to 8.5 percent of all American males (Achenbaum, 1978a: 61, 91). By 1991 the gender gap had widened to 14.7 percent and 10.4 percent, respectively (Schick and Schick, 1994: 7). More significant has been the growing disparity of females to males within the older population. As late as the 1920 federal census, 50.4 percent of all those over 65 were men. Now, there are 69 men for every 100 women among those over the age 65. Men constitute only 16 percent of the nation's centenarians (Yntema, 1997: 188).

The sex differential illustrates gender-specific variations in life expectancy over the life course. The pattern has become more pronounced since 1940. Current life expectancies at birth represent gains of 11.2 years for male babies and 13.6 years for female babies. Women maintain their demographic advantage, albeit in less dramatic terms, after the age of 30. Since 1940, life expectancy at age 65 has increased 5.8 years for women and 3.6 years for men, which translates into a likely death at age 84 for women and 80 for men (Yntema, 1997; Friedland and Summer, 1999: 8). All the evidence points to a fundamental proposition: any institutional changes made to accommodate population aging in the United States must give priority to women's preferences, needs, and capacities.

The elderly population in the United States historically has been white, and it will remain predominantly so in the future. Nonetheless, racial and ethnic variations within the population have become more noticeable over time. At least a fifth of all whites are projected to be over the age of 65 by 2050. The number of blacks over 65 will more than triple during the same period (Dorgan, 1996: 58). The influx of Asians into the United States, especially after World War II, will result in a comparable growth of that subset of the population. Only 6 percent of the Japanese, Chinese, Vietnamese, and other Pacific Islanders were over 65 in 1990. That proportion is expected to rise to 15.3 percent by 2050.

Hispanics, a broad category of people with roots in Spanish-speaking countries, have become a significant and increasingly powerful constituency of the U.S. population in recent decades (Torres-Gil and Kuo, 1998). Indeed, more than half of the foreign-born residents counted in the 2000 census migrated from Latin America. Whereas Italy was the leading country of birth among the foreign born in 1960, Mexico has surpassed all other nations of origin since then. Because most immigrants are young, they are expected to be the fastest-growing segment of the elderly population. Only 5.1 percent of all Hispanics were over 65 in 1990; the percentage will increase to 14.1 percent by 2050. Only 91,000 Hispanics over 85 were enumerated in the 1990 census, but that number is expected to rise to 2.6 million by 2050 (Torres-Gil and Kuo; Hobbs and Damon, 1996: 2-17; Russell, 2003: 318).

The ethnic and racial heterogeneity already visible among the new faces of aging will become more evident over time. Each successive generation is more diverse than the one preceding it. Among men and women between the ages of 15 and 34, Hispanics now outnumber African Americans. Whether they choose to grow old in the United States is not certain: at least 11 percent of all Hispanics are not U.S. citizens, and many may return to their place of birth. But if they do stay here, they will constitute a larger share of the composition of the U.S. older population than at present. Two-thirds of all young adults are non-Hispanic whites, compared to 86 percent of those over the age of 75 (S. Mitchell, 2001: 236–37). To the extent that Hispanic groups conserve inherited values and customs in seeking medical assistance and providing support for elderly kin, we may anticipate that the range of care that rising generations offer their elders will become more ethnically diverse in the twenty-first century. Already the Latinization associated with societal aging is a key factor in the political debates over financing retirement and Social Security (Torres-Gil, 1999).

Economic Trends

The longevity revolution has not increased the number of years that Americans spend in the workforce. Quite the contrary: there has been a long-term decline in labor force participation, particularly among men. According to the 1890 federal census, the first census that offered reliable nationwide age-specific data on occupational patterns, nearly three-quarters of all U.S. males over 65 were gainfully employed. Approximately 60 percent of these workers were farmers, fishers, or miners. About 12 percent of elderly men were working in the industrial sector, 7.3 percent in domestic or personal service, and 6 percent in trade or transportation. Less than 3 percent practiced medicine and law or were teachers or ministers.

Older men's occupational patterns diverged from younger workers' status in two ways in 1890. First, unlike younger workers, older workers sought employment in "traditional" fields as long as possible. Although more than 70 percent of American males were farmers in 1820, seventy years later the proportion had declined to 42 percent. However, farming remained the chief occupation for older workers well into the twentieth century. There were, moreover, notable differences in positions held *within* occupational categories. To cite a dramatic example: less than 6 percent of all professional men were clergy in 1890, but a quarter of all older professional males were ministers. A quarter of all U.S. clergy, according to the 1890 census, were over the age of 65.

Age-specific distinctions appeared in the trades as well as the transportation sectors of the economy as technological and managerial innovations diminished the value of the skills possessed by men over 65. Older tradespeople tended in 1890 to be collectors, shopkeepers, or hucksters. Younger men, on the other hand, sought positions as salespeople, managers, bookkeepers, clerks, and copyists—jobs abundant in an economy that was becoming more bureaucratic and dependent on a new set of skills (Wiebe, 1967; Haber and Gratton, 1994: 98; Achenbaum, 1978: 68). Men under the age of 65 worked as locomotive engineers or other positions associated with building rails and equipment; elderly workers employed by railroad companies served as agents and collectors.

Second, men over the age of 65 were less likely than younger workers to be gainfully employed. Several factors account for the drop-off. Declining health and disability limited older men's opportunities to find positions that were physically demanding. Changes in the marketplace made it more difficult for older workers to stay employed. Machines that depended on interchangeable parts and unskilled labor increasingly eliminated jobs once filled by skilled craftspeople. As industrial and manufacturing concerns established goals based on producing a certain output of goods within a set period of time, managers perceived younger workers to be more efficient than their elders. Commercial enterprises set educational standards for recruits that gave an advantage to younger men with more years of schooling than mature men typically possessed. Seasonal layoffs, depressions and recessions, bankruptcies, and corporate reorganizations all had a more deleterious effect on older than on younger workers. Older workers tended to be unemployed for a longer period of time and sometimes had to settle for becoming janitors or security guards (Achenbaum, 1978: 67; Haber and Gratton, 1994: 98).

The twentieth century saw a dramatic exodus of older male workers from the labor force. The percentage of all men over 65 who were gainfully employed declined 11 percent between 1900 and 1920. During the Great Depression more than a third of all elderly men lost their jobs, compared to a national unemployment rate of 25 percent. Between 1940 and 1993, the proportion of older men who were gainfully employed dropped to 18 percent. Furthermore, there has been a significant increase in the drop-off rate in employment between older and middle-aged workers over time. In 1900, the ratio of the percentage of all men over 65 who were working to the percentage of males gainfully employed between the ages of 45 and 64 was 77 percent. Seventy years later, the ratio was 28 percent (Achenbaum, 1978: 95–103; Hobbs and Damon, 1996: 4-1).

Men over 65 are not the only segment of the population retiring in greater numbers. Men still in their prime also choose to retire early. Changes in Social Security laws in 1961 enabled men to retire at 62 with an actuarial reduction in the benefits they otherwise would have received at age 65. Some men opt to draw on their Individual Retirement Accounts when they reach age 59 and a half (Achenbaum, 1986: 108). As a result, the average age of retirement is no longer 65. In 1950, 87 percent of men between the ages of 55 and 64 were gainfully employed; in 1996, only 67 percent of men in that age range were in the labor force. Some economists doubt that this trend will continue indefinitely, however. They forecast that baby boomers, already worried about the prospects of receiving Social Security benefits, are less likely than their elders to benefit from generous corporate pensions or to be eligible for retiree healthcare coverage from their employers (Yntema, 1997: 134).

The history of older women's career patterns in the twentieth century reflects the profound changes that have occurred in employment opportunities for U.S. women of all ages. Regardless of nativity and ethnicity, most women worked at home at the beginning of the century. Although women constituted 48.8 percent of the total elderly population in 1890, fewer than 10 percent of all older people enumerated by the census as gainfully employed were female. Older women were less likely than middle-aged women to work outside of the home. Younger females tended to work as servants, sales clerks, telephone operators, typists, or teachers. Older women (typically widowed) were more often counted by census takers as lodging-house keepers, seamstresses, practical nurses, or bar keepers. Like their male counterparts, older women had difficulty securing employment in jobs in mills, shoe or knitting industries, or other places where new machines and methods diminished the value of skills females perfected in managing households. Although some institutions enrolled women over the age of 30 to be trained as nurses and doctors, the medical establishment for the most part set age and sex barriers, as did the legal profession (Achenbaum, 1978: 66–69; Haber and Gratton, 1994: 99–100).

The proportion of all employed women working in clerical positions rose from 3.1 percent in 1890 to 20.9 percent in 1930. Forty years later,

34.5 percent of all women in the labor force served as clerical workers. But secretarial work and bookkeeping remained a young female's field: only 2.3 percent of all clerical workers were over 65. To be a good secretary required competence in the latest office technology; many older workers did not and could not adapt.

The exodus of older women from the labor force has not been as dramatic as that of men; it has fluctuated around 10 percent for most of the century. The constancy of this figure stands in marked contrast to the profound increase in the proportion of women, including those with young children, who work outside of the home. The proportion of females of all ages who are gainfully employed increased from 18.2 percent in 1890 to nearly 60 percent today. Examining trends cohort by cohort suggests that the proportion of older women who may seek employment might increase in years ahead. The proportion of women in their thirties who worked outside of the home nearly doubled between 1957 and 1993 as their last child entered day care or school. A similar trend obtains among women in late-middle-age. In 1950 less than a third of all females between 50 and 54 were in the marketplace; the proportion rose to 47 percent in 1970 and to 70 percent in 1993. For the group between 55 and 59, the corresponding percentages are no less striking. The proportion of employed women between the ages of 60 and 64 rose from 21 percent in 1950 to 36 percent twenty years later, but the figure has not much changed since then (Hobbs and Damon, 1996: 4-2; U.S. Department of Labor, 2003).

In short, while it is true that a smaller proportion of older women than older men participate in the labor force, they represent a larger percentage of the labor force than ever before (Smith, 1979). This is because many men are choosing to leave the work force at earlier and earlier ages. Perhaps more important, thanks to changes in employment practices that make allowances for women's responsibilities to their children and to a modest closing of the wage gap, more women are participating longer in the labor force. Some, to be sure, have no choice. They need a regular paycheck to make ends meet. Others want to work long enough to become vested in employer-sponsored healthcare, disability, and retirement benefits.

Employment patterns among minorities vary by ethnic group, gender, and age. To illustrate: in agriculture, a greater percentage of African Americans than whites were farmers between 1890 and 1940. Because of their concentration in farming and need to eke out a living, a greater proportion of older blacks than whites remained in the labor force. Native-born Americans were more likely to be engaged in agricultural pursuits than foreign-born citizens. Race also made a difference in land ownership. Throughout the period whites tended to be owners or managers; the percentage of African-American farm owners did not exceed the percentage of black tenants until 1940 (Achenbaum, 1978: 76, 97).

Amid the dissimilarities that persist across ethnic lines loom gender differences, but with few exceptions, they are not as profound as one might anticipate (Hobbs and Damon, 1996: 4-3). Between 1950 and 1990, white males between the ages of 50 and 70 had higher labor-force participation rates than African-American males because on average the latter group had poorer health, chronic disabilities, and lower educational qualifications. The gap between white males and men of Hispanic origin between 1970 and 1990 was smaller. Over the age of 80, the three groups of men had similar work records. Although after World War II African-American women over the ages of 50 were far more likely than white females to be working, by 1990, the differences in rates were negligible. A strikingly smaller proportion of women of Hispanic origin under the age of 65 were in the labor force in 1990. Over the age of 80, the differences were trivial because fewer than 4 percent of each ethnic group worked.

These data suggest that the historical working/not-working dichotomy among elderly people in the United States is changing. Over time larger percentages of white men in successive cohorts have stopped full-time employment when they have sufficient funds to retire or are physically incapable of continuing in their full-time positions. But some older white men, as well as other segments of the aging population, want to remain in the labor force. Many of them need to supplement their financial resources with gainful employment. For people who want to enjoy the benefits of retirement while still earning some income flexible options exist.

Only 11 percent of all gainfully employed men work part-time, but the percentages increase with age. One out of every five men over the age of 55 works part-time. The figure rises to 48 percent among those over 65. A majority (56%) of men over 75 who are earning wages are working part-time. The percentages are even greater for women. Roughly one in four women in the labor force is working part-time. Among those over

55, the proportion rises to 35 percent. Almost two-thirds of all women over 65 who work do so on a part-time basis. Some of these elderly part-timers are employed a few hours a day or a couple of hours per week. Others take on full-time jobs during holiday seasons or other times of the year (Yntema, 1997: 153).

The Bureau of Labor Statistics defines another set of part-time employees as "alternative" workers—men and women who serve as independent contractors, on-call workers, or temporary-help employees recruited by employment agencies or contract firms. Older Americans are more likely than younger workers to be included in this category. Mature workers are more likely than their younger counterparts to be on call; they prefer to serve as substitute teachers rather than to be temps, because that arrangement better suits their schedule (Yntema, 1997: 157).

Some full-time workers seek some leeway as to when they begin and end their work day. Nearly a fifth of all male workers over 65 report that they have more flexibility in their schedules than their younger counterparts. According to 1991 data, 14.1 percent of all full-time female workers over 65 enjoy flexible work schedules—a figure comparable to the percentages of women between the ages of 25 and 44, who presumably have home-care responsibilities (Dorgan, 1996: 518).

The trend toward part-time and alternative employment among men and women who are already drawing retirement income will likely increase over time. Social Security since the 1940s has become the major source of income in old age. In 1992 it provided at least 50 percent of the funds available to 63 percent of all beneficiaries. No segment of the senior-citizen population underestimates Social Security's importance as a source of retirement income (Hobbs and Damon, 1996: 4-14; Cutler, Whitelaw, and Beattie, 2002: 25). But recipients report that additional earnings make a difference in older Americans' sense of financial security. Money ranked after health as a serious problem among those surveyed in the 2000 National Council on Aging's *American Perceptions of Aging in the Twenty-first Century* (Cutler, Whitelaw, and Beattie: 3). Thirty-six percent of those over 65 worry about having enough financial resources for the rest of their lives. Women are more concerned than men. African Americans are twice as anxious as whites. Those with less education worry more than college graduates.

Money concerns are reflected in spending patterns. Households headed by men and women in retirement buy roughly one-third less than the typical U.S. household, in part because they have smaller household sizes. They spend more on certain items—prescription drugs, health insurance, appliances, and charities—than the average household. It is worth noting, however, that even in prosperous times like the 1990s, elderly people were not the only ones who kept track of their expenditures. Between 1990 and 1997, householders aged 35 to 44 cut their spending. In contrast, those between the ages of 45 and 54 maintained their reputation for being hearty consumers, if not invariably big spenders. All of this suggests that the state of the economy and each cohort's sense of its vulnerability play as large a role in perceptions of economic well-being as does the actual wealth and income that a particular age group possesses.

Healthful Longevity

Health concerned more senior citizens interviewed (42%) than money (36%) in the 2000 survey by the National Council on the Aging (NCOA). Baby boomers were less worried about health than those over 65, but there were differences within the elderly population. Women, blacks, those who did not graduate from high school, and persons over 75 were more inclined than their peers to say that health was a "very or somewhat serious" problem (Cutler, Whitelaw, and Beattie, 2002: 3). Health problems played a greater role than "not having enough money" in the decision to retire completely (ibid.: 21).

Without discounting the opinions and fears of America's old persons, it must be quickly added that those whom NCOA surveyed in 2000 were more optimistic in assessing their health than the cohort in 1974 reported. There was a 12 percent decline in the proportion of persons claiming that health was a "serious personal problem" in that twenty-six-year period. Racial differences were greater than gender differences, but the gap between blacks and whites was wider in 1974 than in 2000 (ibid.: 2, 72–73). Those between the ages of 50 and 59 saying that their health was good or excellent rose, according to a government survey, from 63 percent to 80 percent between 1974 to 1980 (Russell, 2003: 96). Experts reason that this is partly due to the increasingly higher levels of educational attainment across rising cohorts: better-educated people tend to be more health conscious and to take steps to stay in shape and watch their diet.

Indeed, there is considerable evidence that today's elderly, baby boomers, and those in the cohort behind them are taking preventive measures to maintain their health. Giving up smoking has been proven to be beneficial at every age in reducing the risks of lung, breast, and bladder cancers and heart disease. Between 1925 and 1992 the proportion of all men over 65 who smoked dropped to 16 percent, whereas the percentage of older women smokers rose to 12 percent during the same period. That more than a third of all black elders smoke accounts for much of their respiratory difficulties (Manheimer, 1994: 380–81; Hobbs and Damon, 1996: 3-15).

Older people are more inclined than younger ones to report that they watch their diet, opting for "healthy heart diets" (Yntema, 1997: 62–63). Americans of all ages are eating differently from decades ago—though increased consumption of fat undercuts the salutary effects of some of their prudent choices. Older Americans as a group report less alcohol consumption (and more abstention) than any other age group; in contrast, roughly a third of all those between 18 and 30 engage in binge drinking (ibid.: 65; S. Mitchell, 2001: 103). Exercise plays a greater role in daily living for most Americans. Males in their thirties and forties are the most likely age group to run or swim or play sports at least twice a week; women their age have lower rates of participation (S. Mitchell, 84). Few mobile older people are "couch potatoes": senior citizen centers and YMCAs provide older people opportunities to do yoga and calisthenics and to stay limber.

As a result of greater health consciousness, preventive measures, and advances in medicine, surgery, and pharmacology, older men and women tend to succumb to different causes of death from their forbears. In 1900 elderly people were likely to die from pneumonia, infectious diseases, or industrial accidents. Heart disease has been the leading cause of death (33 percent among those over 65, 44 percent among those over 85) in recent decades, though there has been a decline in its prevalence since the 1960s. Cancer is the second leading killer, but remarkable progress has been made in curing the disease. Only 20 percent of those diagnosed with cancer survived five years in the 1960s; the figure has doubled since then. Strokes are the third cause of death; their incidence doubles every five years among those over 60. Next come chronic obstructive pulmonary disease, pneumonia, and deaths from a multitude of causes. Alzheimer's disease, unidentified until the early twentieth century, is now an important cause of death in late life whose significance is expected to grow over time (Hobbs and Damon, 1996: 3-9, 3-11). In contrast, those between the ages of 15 and 34 are most likely to die violently from accidents or murder. AIDS was the second leading cause of death among the young, though new treatments have prolonged lives (S. Mitchell, 2001: 117).

Significant improvements have been made in mortality rates by preventing or controlling acute diseases. The current cohort of older Americans feels healthier than their predecessors. But not all reports about healthful longevity are good. The incidence of chronic ailments has become more prevalent as men and women live longer. Disability with advancing age represents the modern-day equivalent of the fate of Tithonos: worsening health typically accompanies a longer expected life, particularly over the age of 80. Seventy percent of all octogenarian women and 53 percent of all men over 80 had at least two chronic complaints, including visual or hearing impairment, hypertension, varicose veins, strokes, or some form of depression (Hobbs and Damon, 1996: 3-17). Disabilities and chronic illnesses are likely to emerge among men and women in their prime and then persist for the rest of their lives. Less than one in seven suffers a disability between the ages of 22 to 44; one in four between the ages of 45 and 54 has a disability (Russell, 1999: 107). Those who survive heart attacks in their fifties may spend the rest of their lives coping with limitations in mobility and functioning, not to mention living with the fear that the next attack will be fatal. American medicine, which has been so successful in conquering acute disease, must now grapple with an aging population likely to be afflicted with minor chronic ailments and major disabilities.

It is important to underline the gender difference in mortality and morbidity rates in the U.S. population. Women live longer than men; they are also more likely to report health or physical problems. Females can anticipate enduring more years of physical dependency than males. More women over the age of 65 (10%) than older men report difficulty in walking, though problems with mobility for both sexes almost double between the ages of 75 and 84 (Hobbs and Damon, 1996: 3-21). The same differential applies to getting outside, bathing, eating, dressing, and using the toilet. Only in one instance—using the telephone—do men over 65 and men over 85 report greater difficulty than their female peers. Functional limitations, moreover, are greater among blacks than whites. About 60 percent of all African Americans over 65 had one or more functional limitations, according to a 1991 survey, compared to 50 percent of all whites over 65 (Hobbs and Damon, 1996: 3-20).

The need for assistance in performing everyday activities, consequently, increases with age. Less than 3 percent of all Americans between the ages of 15 and 64 require aid. Roughly one in ten of men and women between the ages of 65 and 74 who are not in nursing homes need help. Over the age of 75, 22.8 percent of all men and 32.9 percent of all women require aid. Most older people remain at home, but the likelihood of entering a nursing home increases with age—in 1990 soaring to nearly a quarter of those over 85. Most of these residents were women, who constitute one-third of all people living in nursing homes (Hobbs and Damon, 1996: 6-9).

Chronicity, leading to diminishing capacity over time and (for a significant minority of elders) institutionalization at advanced age, is not new, but it represents an increasingly visible facet of aging. Diagnosing ailments that present differently later in the life course is bound to be an increasingly important aspect of medical practice. Unfortunately, Americans' confidence in medicine—along with government, press, and education—has declined in recent years. The decline between 1974 and 2000 is less apparent among those over 70 than in any other age group (Russell, 2003: 32). But elderly people have some basis for skepticism: roughly a quarter of all senior citizens were prescribed sedatives, antidepressants, analgesics, and other medications, "drugs that they should almost never take" (Dorgan, 1996: 336). Some older people over-medicate with drugs that they no longer need or that should not be taken in combination with other medicines. Educating older adults to be their own caregivers will become an increasingly important societal priority.

Activating Potentials beyond the Marketplace

Researchers demonstrate that education plays a critical role in active longevity. "Education extends both total life expectancy and active life expectancy. Education may thus serve as a powerful social protective mechanism delaying the onset of health problems at older ages" (quoted in Hobbs and Damon, 1996: 6-15). If this is so, it is reasonable to predict that the quest for vital aging will be facilitated by the fact that on average each cohort of elderly men and women will be better educated than the preceding cohort. There has been a sharp rise in the educational attainments of today's older Americans because they had greater access to high-school education than their parents. Nearly three-quarters of all whites over 55 have completed secondary school. Even so, the current cohort of elderly people are the least-educated segment of the population in terms of schooling at all levels (Yntema, 1997: v, 53).

As the baby boomers enter late life, they bring with them even more impressive credentials. Roughly a third of all men aged 50 to 54 in 1999 had earned at least a bachelor's degree, a percentage greater than that achieved by persons between the ages of 35 and 54. Younger adults, on the other hand, are more likely than their elders to pursue their college education on a part-time basis. Insofar as highly educated people tend to seek more learning, experts predict that boomers will head for campuses in their fifties and sixties. Although participation in adult education activities declines with age, the proportion of men and women taking nondegree courses for basic skills and personal development rose modestly between 1995 and 1999 (Russell, 1999: 53, 55, 63, 65; S. Mitchell, 2001: 69).

Racial and ethnic differences, especially among younger Americans, are worth underscoring. Fully 93 percent of all Asian Americans between the ages of 25 and 34 were high-school graduates in 2000. Half of all Asian Americans of that age group have earned at least a bachelor's degree. Thanks to greater opportunities for African Americans, 89 percent of those between the ages of 25 and 34 are high-school graduates; less than half, however, attended college, and only 18 percent earned a degree. Hispanic Americans are the least likely to have completed high school (59%), and only 9 percent have earned college degrees. This disparity is not likely to change much because many younger Hispanics are immigrants with little prior formal schooling (S. Mitchell, 2001: 58; Yntema, 1997: 53).

Educational attainments by gender have changed over time. Men once were more likely than women to complete their college degrees. By the 1999–2000 academic year, women earned considerably more associate, bachelor, and master's degrees than men. Baby boomer women are more likely than men their age to be enrolled in classes. Once again, Hispanics lag behind other ethnic groups (Russell, 1999: 60, 63; Russell, 2003: 76).

Reasons for pursuing adult education vary by age. More than 70 percent of those between the ages of 25 and 54 surveyed in 1995 took courses to enhance their chances for advancement on the job or to train for a new position. Those over 55 reported that they took a course in some educational setting as a way to attain personal growth or to find social interactions—a viewpoint more frequently expressed by those advanced in years (Russell, 1999: 67). Learning for its own sake appeals to the present cohort of older Americans; there is no reason to suspect that younger cohorts will forego educational opportunities when they grow older.

The same pattern obtains for volunteering. Although statistics vary, rates of volunteering have been increasing over time for young and old alike. More than a quarter of all Americans over age 75 volunteer their time (Manheimer, 1994: 758; Dorgan, 1996: 7). Volunteering is a way for people of all ages to contribute to society and to interact with others. The upward trend is bound to continue. According to the latest survey by the National Council on the Aging (Cutler, Whitelaw, and Beattie, 2002: 59), baby boomers are twice as likely as those over 65 (85% compared to 42%) to do volunteer work.

Aging, Religion, and Spirituality

Much of the volunteer effort of elderly people benefits religious institutions. The United States is the most religious nation among advanced industrial countries if its citizens accurately report their religious views and practices. A majority of all Americans over 25 surveyed in 1994 said that they had no doubts that God exists, and those between the ages of 55 and 64 are the most pious (Russell, 1999: 37). That said, religious differences between younger and older cohorts are widening. Those between 18 and 24 express the most reservations of any age group about an Ultimate Reality; a quarter of this group does not express any specific religious preferences. Those between 25 and 34 rank second in nonaffiliation. This does not portend that the United States may someday become a nation of atheists. Rather, it reflects the fact that younger people are inclined to mix the beliefs and practices of various faith traditions, including those from the East; their elders are more likely to consider themselves Roman Catholic, Protestant, or Jewish (S. Mitchell, 2001: 34–35).

Older Americans, moreover, are more predisposed to attend religious services and to pray regularly than younger cohorts. Most of those between the ages of 50 and 59 attend services at least once a month; 61 percent report that they pray daily—though the percentage participating in services declines slightly among those over the age of 60. Because most Christian denominations emphasize the ideal of its congregants to attain "maturity, to the measure of the full stature of Christ" (Ephesians 4:13, NRSV), it is ironic that mainstream denominations provide little instruction or age-based religious rituals for older congregants. Like Jewish communities, Christians celebrate rites of passage at birth, in adolescence, and at marriage (Achenbaum, 1995: 206; Dorgan, 1996: 7; Yntema, 1997: 31). Such data suggest to some researchers that institutionalized religion may lose some of its luster in the decades ahead, especially if young people do not (re)join mainline faith communities in order to provide their children with religious education and age-based rites of passage.

Over the past several decades, gerontologists have paid attention to the increasing manifestations of spirituality, especially among older Americans. Two-thirds of all senior citizens who responded to the National Council on the Aging survey (Cutler, Whitelaw, and Beattie, 2002: 56) reported that only enjoying family and friends and good health surpassed having a rich spiritual life in contributing to a meaningful vital life. There has been an outpouring of books arguing that spiritual well-being contributes directly or indirectly to healthy aging through enhanced social support and better hygienic practices (Koenig, 1995: 24–25). Although scientists dispute some of the claims made for spirituality's efficacy in this realm, there is evidence that those older people who can look deeply within themselves as well as see their place on this vast planet are able to come to terms with dying and death better than those who are less self-reflective. And while primary attention has been placed on the spiritual connections to aging, there is considerable evidence that spiritual awakening is likely to occur earlier, in midlife. Through practice and self-development, those who tap their spiritual strengths are better prepared to face the joys and vicissitudes that come with advancing years (Atchley, 1995: 71).

Realities and Myths of the Older Americans' Political Clout

Although the proportion of all Americans who voted in presidential elections declined from the 1964 election (69%) through the 1988 election, voter turnout slowly rose after the 1992 election. Throughout this period older people were the most likely of all age groups to cast a ballot. Nearly two-thirds of those over 75 went to the polls. In every election, older men were more likely to vote than older women (Hobbs and Damon, 1996: 6-23). The turnout of elderly people in congressional elections is only slightly lower than that for presidential elections (Dorgan, 1996: 572).

Older people do not cast ballots as a bloc, however. Gender, economic, educational, and social differences affect their vote. Divisions are more apparent within older and younger cohorts than across age lines. Older voters generally vote consistently over their lifetimes. Those who came of age in conservative political eras tend to vote Republican. The trauma of the Depression and the achievements of the New Deal made many young people Democrats, and they have remained loyal to the party since then. Older people tend to be so partisan that they are the least likely to support an Independent candidate (Binstock and Quadagno, 2001: 336).

In contrast, voter turnout is lowest among young adults, although it increases rapidly among the 35–45 age group. Increases thereafter are more gradual, declining only among those of advanced age. In the 1996 election, for instance, men and women over 65 represented only 16.5 percent of the voting population but cast 20.3 percent of the ballots. Less than a third of those between the ages of 18 and 24 voted. The proportions increased to 49 percent among those between the ages of 25 and 44, and 64 percent among those 45 to 64 (ibid.: 334). Part of the difference is due to the lack of propensity among younger people to sign up to vote (though now that some states have made voter registration part of the process of obtaining a driver's license, the gap may narrow).

Younger and older voters differ in at least two other ways. On the one hand, young adults in 1998 were more likely to identify themselves as political Independents than as Republicans or Democrats. Although federal policy-making has been greatly influenced by neoconservative ideologies since the Vietnam War, those young adults who do identify with a party generally attach themselves (though not consistently) with the Democratic rather than the Republican party. Older voters on average are slightly more likely to support conservative positions and less likely to opt for liberal viewpoints—even though 43 percent of those over 65 considered themselves Democrats, the remainder dividing fairly equally between Republicans and Independents (S. Mitchell, 2001: 37–39). Furthermore, men and women over 60 tend to express more confidence in the federal government than do younger people—though they claimed in 1994 to have slightly less confidence in Congress than the rest of the population (Yntema, 1997: 44–45).

Since the 1980s, older people have often been caricatured in the media as "greedy geezers." Conservatives argue that "generational inequity" has become a major political issue. They claim that the elderly population's entitlements have become too costly, that older Americans who collect Social Security, Medicare, and other benefits are squandering the future resources that are due to rising generations (Peterson, 1999). Demographers, policy analysts, and economists have systematically challenged this perspective. Apparently, they have been somewhat successful because according to the most recent National Council on Aging survey (Cutler, Whitelaw, and Beattie, 2002: 66), less than 15 percent of the population thinks the elderly population wields too much political influence. (Curiously, those over 65 are slightly more inclined to hold this view than are young people or baby boomers.) The myth of grandparents living high off the hog in Florida while children go hungry remains prevalent in the media, however.

Family and Friends: Keys to Vital Aging

The "ideal" family structure, most Americans assume, is a "little commonwealth" consisting of a mother and father and their children living in a single household. Marriage is key to this picture. An overwhelming majority of all married couples in every age group over the age of 18 consider themselves "very" happy or "pretty" happy in their relationships (Russell, 1999: 24). That said, household arrangements suggest a more complex picture. Nuclear families represent only a quarter of all household situations. The percentage of individuals living alone in the United States rose dramatically in the twentieth century; 31 percent of all households in 2000 consisted of people living alone or with nonrelatives. The proportion of married couples heading households in the U.S. population fell from 78 percent in 1950 to 53 percent in 2000 (Russell, 2003: 276). The reasons for the decline in the percentage of nuclear family households vary by age cohort.

Among those between the ages of 65 and 74 in 1993, a higher proportion of men and women are living alone. Only 24 percent of people over the age of 85 in 1993 lived with a spouse, and 48 percent lived alone. Nearly twice as many elderly men as women were married. Elderly women were more than three times as likely as elderly men to be widowed in 1993. Five percent of older men and women who were divorced had not remarried (Hobbs and Damon, 1996: 6-1).

It is little wonder, then, that older people put such value on friendship, especially relationships of several decades' duration. Nursing home residents report having up to six close friends with whom they interact at least several times a month (Manheimer, 1994: 346–47). According to the 2000 National Council on the Aging report (Cutler, Whitelaw, and Beattie, 2002: 56), nearly nine out of ten elderly respondents declared that having close relationships with friends and family was key to a meaningful, rich life—a slightly higher percentage than was attributed to taking care of one's health. Besides warding off feelings of isolation and loneliness, such bonds, in the minds of older respondents, made them "warm and friendly." Although researchers do not think that friends promote psychological well-being as efficaciously as does marriage, having a number of intimate companions is beneficial nonetheless (ibid.: 7; Hobbs and Damon, 1996: 6-5).

Married couples dominated the households of those aged 35 to 54 in 1993. Seventy percent of all couples in this cohort who had lived together at least five years eventually married. But many boomers postpone marriage or choose never to marry. Divorce is prevalent: the per capita rate quadrupled between 1970 and 1996 (*Divorce Reform*, 2003). Half of all first marriages of men under 45 end in divorce; for baby boomer women's first marriages the proportion is slightly higher. Children of broken marriages typically live with their mothers. Women in this cohort head 32 percent of black households, compared to 20 percent of the Hispanic and 11 percent of the white households. The effect of late marriage, no marriage, or divorce and separation on African-American households can be inferred from the fact that only 8 percent of all black women between the ages of 35 and 39 live alone (Russell, 1999: 190).

Marriages among baby boomers are especially susceptible to divorce in the first ten years. Cumulatively, half of all of their first marriages ended in divorce, and so do 60 percent of their remarriages. In 1997 the median length of a marriage was 7.2 years. Men were on average 36 at their first divorce; women, 33 according to *Divorce Magazine* (2003). In addition, baby boomer women can expect to experience widowhood at an older age than their mothers, given advances in adult longevity. That said, they probably will also experience widowhood or being divorced for a longer duration of their later years (Hobbs and Damon, 1996: 6-5).

The experiences of Generation X, aged 18 to 34 in 2001, provide another set of cohort-specific living arrangements. This group was slightly
less likely than older cohorts to have been living with both parents when
they were 16. Three-quarters of those over 55 had been raised by two
parents, compared to 51 percent of the younger set. The death of a parent accounts for 54 percent of the single families for those over the age
of 65. In contrast, 71 percent of those between the ages of 18 and 24
who were living with a single parent were children of divorce (S.
Mitchell, 2003: 11, 13). Generation X has thus far been less likely to
marry than older cohorts. Slightly more than half of all Hispanic and
white women have not been married. The proportion of unmarried black
women between the ages of 15 and 34 is even higher (73%). Young men
are more likely to remain single than young women. Whites are more
likely to be divorced than Hispanics or blacks (ibid.: 224). These marital trends are significant because most babies are born to women between
the ages of 20 and 29. Nowadays one in three babies is born to an unmarried woman, whereas in 1950 only 4 percent were born out of wedlock
(Russell, 2003: 98).

These data corroborate the importance of gender, ethnicity, and race
in studying population aging and indicate that patterns are becoming
more diverse. They also underscore the growing importance of alternative living arrangements, especially among younger cohorts. Non-nuclear
families have increased in importance as younger men and women postpone marriage, middle-aged couples divorce, older women experience
more years of widowhood, and people of all age groups opt to live with
partners outside of marriage (Russell, 2003: xxii).

Researchers on aging prefer longitudinal to cross-sectional data because
they provide an opportunity to track continuities and changes in specific
individuals over their life course. Relying on cross-sectional data con-
founds age, cohort, and period effects. We cannot predict whether a
woman beset with several chronic illnesses at age 40 will be more disabled at 80 than a woman who has no disability. Nor do we know
whether men and women in their twenties are more likely to return to
their parents' homes because of the economy or because prolonging adolescence is becoming a new norm. Extra years of living are bound to alter
the chronological boundaries of the life span, but the data used here cannot tell us when, how, or why.

Unfortunately, there is no longitudinal data set that covers all of the

aging that have been discussed in this chapter. Still, the informa-
ered here about successive cohorts is instructive. The statistics
give us a sense of the current status of various age groups. Insofar as
people act in certain ways at particular stages of life, the data enable us
to make provisional speculations about the future needs and predispo-
sitions of the U.S. population that its institutions must accommodate.

Since World War II, six major trends have transformed American
society (see also Russell, 2003: xxii). First, Americans on average can
expect to live longer than their parents and grandparents. Their physical and mental conditions vary with added years. That they differ from
the status of younger people will force healthcare providers to pay at
least as much attention to disability and chronicity as to acute illness in
the second half of life. Second, not only have women's life expectancies
expanded more than men's, but females' roles in the marketplace, at
home, and in various religious and social institutions have also broad-
ened. Women are going to play an increasingly more prominent part in
shaping the contours of societal aging. Third, the U.S. population has
grown more diverse and tolerant as blacks, Hispanics, and Asians increase in numbers and power. With generational succession, the older
segments of the population will be less white. Fourth, with the growing
acceptance of divorce and of people who choose to live alone, nuclear
households no longer predominate. Alternative living arrangements will
undoubtedly become common as Generation X grows older. Fifth, each
successive cohort of Americans has attained more years of education.
The education boom should have an effect on the nation's health and
productivity. Finally, because the United States has enjoyed more prosperous than lean years since World War II, a greater proportion of the
U.S. population enjoys economic security than ever before in our history.

Economic growth and continued gains in productivity will make it
easier for the nation to come to terms with the benefits and challenges
of population aging (Friedland and Summer, 1999); however, Americans will have to modify many institutional arrangements to capitalize
on the assets of the older population. And if economic growth is more
important than demographic trends in ensuring continued prosperity,
then we need clearer images of the psychological profiles and functional
potentials of late life (Qualls and Abeles, 2000: 4).

The New Age of Production and Consumption } 2

In the depths of the Great Depression, Dr. Frances Townsend galvanized so many older citizens with his proposals to restore prosperity that for a while his movement seemed poised to transform the U.S. political landscape. Townsend's earlier careers hardly prepared him to emerge as a radical leader. He had practiced medicine in the Midwest until he moved to Long Beach, California, in 1919. To supplement his meager practice, Townsend ventured into real estate, but his timing was bad. The bottom was falling out of the housing market. Townsend then accepted a position in the city's health bureau. When funds for public employees dried up, he had to go on relief. On January 1, 1934, Dr. Townsend created a nonprofit corporation, Old Age Revolving Pensions, Ltd., to get folks like him (then aged 67), who knew firsthand the tragedy of being old and poor, out of their desperate straits. The plan, he believed, would also revive the nation's economy (Neuberger and Loe, 1936: 31–32).

Old Age Revolving Pensions, Ltd., had three components. First, all U.S. citizens age 60 and older were to receive $200 per month if they met two conditions: that they not seek work, and that they spend the pension within thirty days. Second, the U.S. government would print $2 billion in currency to get the new money in circulation. Third, a 2 percent sales tax on all business transactions was to finance the old-age pensions thereafter. The plan appealed to elders. By December 1934 there were 500,000 dues-paying members of Townsend Clubs all over the country (Foner and Garraty, 1991: 1080). A year later there were 7,000 clubs with a total membership conservatively estimated at 1.5 million older men and women (Holtzman, 1975: 75).

Diehard followers believed that Dr. Townsend's panacea was divinely inspired, but elements of the plan probably had their incarnation elsewhere. Advertising executive Bruce Barton, proposing to "let the young do the work and old men loaf," recommended in the August 1931 issue of *Vanity Fair* that men retire at age 45 on half salary (quoted in Putnam, 1970: 50). That same year, four years before New Dealers enacted legislation to reduce old-age poverty, journalist Stuart McCord suggested that President Roosevelt might end the Depression with an old-age pension system financed by a national sales tax. McCord proposed annuities of $50–80 a month to those who retired at 50 or 55 (Putnam, 1970: 50–51; Holtzman, 1975: 34). American writer and activist Upton Sinclair and Governor Huey Long wanted to give Americans over 60 pensions worth, respectively, $30 and $50 a month as part of their utopian schemes to redistribute the nation's wealth.

Townsend intended to grant senior citizens $200 a month ($50 more than he had in mind in 1933) "so that no one would come along and offer more" (quoted in Holtzman, 1975: 38). Besides its psychological appeal, Dr. Townsend realized the sum's significant economic value. Because the Great Depression, in his opinion, was caused by overproduction, it could be cured by increasing consumption dramatically. Distancing himself from both Sinclair and Long, Townsend denied that his plan "soaked the rich." Furthermore, unlike New Dealers who put their trust in an alphabet of agencies, Townsend felt that his plan could abolish old-age poverty and restore prosperity without necessitating a cumbersome bureaucracy. He viewed the federal government's role as oversight.

Dr. Townsend's plan made its way to Congress on several occasions. Townsendites lobbied hard, but the numbers did not add up. Among other things, experts warned lawmakers that the 2 percent tax was not enough to finance the program. Worse, the tax might ruin businesses struggling to recover. Jobs vacated by elders probably would be abolished rather than filled by young people, according to economists, so there would be no net reduction in unemployment. Lawmakers understandably worried that collecting a new tax and then distributing money to senior citizens would be difficult and expensive to do. Dr. Townsend's vagueness during congressional testimonies, especially about the sales tax, hardly helped his cause. Independent studies by think tanks such as the Twentieth Century Fund demonstrated that the plan was "dangerously unworkable" (Schneider, 1937: viii; see also Twentieth Century Fund on Old Age Security, 1936). Townsendites nevertheless goaded the Roosevelt administration to deal with the plight of older Americans. Even the enactment of the Social Security Act in 1935 did not immediately derail the Townsendite crusade. Proponents lobbied Congress for modified versions of the Townsend Plan until the movement lost most of its momentum by 1940.

Actuarial flaws and unrealistic economic assumptions doomed the plan as a policy instrument for ending the Great Depression. Yet Dr. Townsend's characterizations of older people as (non)producers, as consumers, and as a homogeneous age-based constituency still have some currency today. It is worth examining continuities and changes in these three late-life roles since the 1930s.

First, personal observation convinced Francis Townsend that most of his contemporaries devalued the contributions that older persons could make to society. Dr. Townsend was not alone in his critique. Consider Corra Harris's description of old people as "The Borrowed Timers" in the September 1926 issue of *Ladies Home Journal:* "Old people are not so much prisoners of their years and their infirmities as they are of their circumstances, after they are no longer able to produce their own circumstances, but are obliged to adjust themselves to conditions made for them by people who belong to a later generation in a new world. It is worse than if they became foreigners in their old age, because they are in the midst of familiar scenes, but obsolete, like fine words erased from the epic of living" (C. Harris, 1926: 35).

The 1920 census indicated that, as the percentage of men and women over 65 in the population grew, the proportion of elderly men in the labor force was declining—even in the agricultural sector, where most found their livelihood. When the skills of older craftspeople grew obsolescent in the industrial sector, aged workers were replaced by machines and by younger people with better training. Hiring and transferring practices discriminated against men over 40. Those with gray hair rarely stood a chance of obtaining positions comparable to ones they had lost. Elderly workers had to settle for menial work, occasional jobs, or time on their hands. "In no other country does the basis of age alone furnish so definite a line of demarcation between a portion of the population recognized as economically efficient and socially attractive and that part of it which is neither useful nor particularly attractive" (Dallach, 1933: 50).

Roughly a quarter of the U.S. labor force lost their jobs in the Great Depression. Its impact on older workers was devastating. According to the Massachusetts Census for Unemployment, the average unemployment rate in that commonwealth in 1934 was 25.2 percent (Achenbaum, 1978a: 128). Older people had progressively higher unemployment rates because they were perceived as the least desirable workers. No wonder Townsend stipulated that people over 60 should quit their jobs and collect pensions. Older workers past their prime, he felt, should give way to younger men with families to support.

Once out of work in the Depression, elderly persons could rely on few sources of economic support. Bank foreclosures wiped out their savings. Corporations and trade unions suspended pension plans. Older people's sons and daughters had enough difficulty taking care of their children without being burdened with caring for their parents. Something had to be done.

Second, older people might assist in the nation's recovery, Dr. Townsend believed, by assuming an unprecedented role as consumers. He saw elders fulfilling a pent-up demand for cars, radios, clothes, and other products. Hardly a handout, which would have been much smaller, a $200 monthly pension would give beneficiaries the wherewithal to "prime the pump." Townsend's notion of older people as productive consumers was well calculated: the United States after World War I had become a consumer-driven nation. "A wide array of commentators, activists, and authorities made Americans acutely aware of their new collective role as consumers. A vast literature—novels, social science monographs, government reports, magazine pieces, trade journal articles, reform tracts—documented and dissected, celebrated and abominated the new culture of consumption" (Fox and Lears, 1983: 103).

The $200 pension, Dr. Townsend knew, far exceeded the $94.75 monthly paycheck that the average U.S. worker earned in 1935 (U.S. Bureau of the Census, 1960: 95). A continuous senior spending spree, he reckoned, would generate jobs for young workers. The pension would help to end the Depression in other ways. Older people's newly gained affluence would eliminate them from the dole. Increased demand for goods was bound to create more job openings for wage-earning heads of household in the manufacturing and service sectors (Putnam, 1970: 53).

Third, Dr. Townsend envisioned that his plan would alter perceptions of older Americans' status. Throughout most of U.S. history, the vicissitudes of growing older were viewed as individual problems, largely handled in the private sphere. With the exception of the Grand Army of the Republic (GAR), no organization had ever served all of the country's elderly citizens—and the GAR pandered mainly to the self-interest of Civil War veterans and their families. Townsend's genius was to encourage millions of older Americans to protest their economic misfortune. He appealed to men and women who, having played by the rules, were now mired in a miserable old age. Mobilizing their resources, Townsendites drew national attention to old-age dependency. Only federal intervention, they emphasized, could alleviate the problem. Patriotism was integral to the campaign; Townsendites wanted to get the nation moving again. The origins of today's "gray lobby" lie in the Townsend Clubs.

As we shall see, recent historical developments have undermined all three of Dr. Townsend's assumptions. Although the average age at which men leave their full-time jobs continues to decline, many seek some sort of employment or engage in a volunteer activity after retirement. The concept of "fixed retirement" at a certain age is changing. And, finally, while no one doubts that older people possess a large share of the nation's wealth, many advertisers ignore "the gray market," appealing instead to the young. Even those who appreciate how much discretionary income older people possess are not sure how to make gold out of gray. The older population constitutes such a diverse group that age-based marketing strategies rarely succeed in reaching their target.

Retiring into "Unretirement"

"Retirement" as an economic institution has changed dramatically over the past half-century. Surveys and scholarly investigations document that older workers have been both "pushed" and "pulled" to leave the labor force at earlier ages. Many do so in their fifties and early sixties, before they become eligible for full Social Security benefits. Retirement patterns among women differ from men's because of the steady influx of women of all ages into the labor pool since the 1940s (see chapter 1).

"Retirement" is a personal milestone that occurs mainly to those in the second half of life. Nonetheless, its eventuality shadows the life course

(Hobbs and Damon, 1996: 4-1; Visser and Beatty, 2003: 9). Middle-aged employees are more inclined than previous cohorts to maximize opportunities by seeking new employment rather than remaining with one firm for decades. Those who have switched jobs often view retirement as just another transition, not the capstone of their careers. Younger people, worried about Social Security and their savings, are beginning to make retirement plans early. "The idea that we will someday retire is increasingly present to all adults and it is even urged on adolescents," notes David Ekerdt (2004: 3). "The earliest reaches of adulthood are being colonized by frequent reminders that it takes individual effort to achieve retirement."

Planning, good health, and luck make for successful retirements. But individuals are not the only actors deciding when and how retirement takes place. Institutional priorities and prejudices affect employees' decisions to leave full-time jobs, while encouraging others to "un-retire" to part-time positions with flexible hours and benefits. A combination of impediments and inducements is altering the dimensions of "normal" retirement. Let us begin by identifying those constraints that have impeded older workers for more than a century, because they continue to affect retirement options.

Businesses and industries have long weighed the costs and benefits of retaining senior employees. For the sake of efficiency, corporate managers in the past discharged those whose productivity was waning (Graebner, 1980). Cost effectiveness has been another consideration; older workers on average are more expensive than young recruits. Long years of service result in higher salaries, greater pension benefits, and higher insurance costs, especially for health coverage. Few seasoned veterans have willingly switched industries if their skills were firm-specific or if they feared loss of benefits by moving on (Bluestone et al., 1990: 283; O. Mitchell, 1993: 65). Sometimes, of course, circumstances give them no choice but to leave their current positions.

Amid the multinational corporate restructuring that reconfigured the U.S. marketplace in the late 1980s, older workers found it harder than younger ones to find other jobs. According to a 1988 survey of the Bureau of Labor Statistics, 82 percent of all displaced workers between the ages of 25 and 54 were re-employed. In contrast, only 60 percent of those between 55 and 64 got jobs, and a mere 35 percent of workers over 64 found new employment (Goldberg, 2000: 54–55). The jobs that displaced older workers obtain, by and large, are less desirable than the ones they held: they pay less and offer fewer amenities, and they tend to be of shorter duration than those available to younger displaced workers (O. Mitchell, 1993: 90–91).

Labor experts agree that ageism is the major factor influencing human resource decisions to discharge older workers. Younger job candidates typically fare better in hiring. Despite the protection afforded by the Age Discrimination in Employment Act, stereotypes about older people's potential usefulness that pervaded the marketplace a century ago still persist. The most damaging "strongly held assumption," claims Beverly Goldberg (2000: 113), "is that older workers are not as creative or productive as younger workers." Employees of a certain age are also considered to be less flexible, less adaptable, and more costly than their junior colleagues. Decades of empirical evidence debunking these negative images have not yet succeeded in overturning the image of older workers as being "over the hill."

Ageism insinuates itself into the organizational structures and policies of corporate America. Performance appraisals that use subjective rating scales generally yield more negative assessments of older workers than criteria that are considered age neutral. Furthermore, intergenerational frictions arise, it is said, when cohort-specific values and styles clash over management issues and objectives (Schaie and Schooler, 1998: 163; Konrad, 2001). Rounding out the psychological barrage against older workers is that age group's presumed fear of mastering new technologies. Human resource managers are reluctant to invest in retooling older workers because of their purported slow learning curve (Goldberg, 2000: 114–18). In addition, health matters play a part. Many employers assume that elderly men and women workers have high absentee rates due to illness. Many elderly employees internalize such negative feedback, discounting their own possible value to their employers (Kim and Moon, 2002).

Ageism has caused structural and cultural lags in the labor force. It is evident in the rather meager efforts corporations make to (re)train older workers. In the past, employees who worked at desks usually maintained their jobs longer than peers whose viability depended on their physical strength. Now aging managers, secretaries, and other white-collar employees are vulnerable if they do not keep abreast of developments in digitalized work content and advances in information technology. The longer an employee has remained in a certain position, the more important training becomes to learn new sets of cognitive tasks (Visser and Beatty, 2003: 9; Schaie and Schooler, 1998: 9). Ageism, of course, is not the only issue determining whether to (re)train aging employees. The size of the work site, for instance, is a factor. Small firms are less likely to offer in-house training in new technologies than larger companies (Bass et al., 1993: 88). But the insidiousness of age-based prejudice is ubiquitous.

That employers have ambivalent feelings about retraining older workers often sets into motion a sequence of events that culminates in discharging members of that age cohort. Human resource managers complain that mature employees lack the skills necessary in an increasingly global economy. The Bureau of Labor Statistics found that workers under 25 or over 55 are less likely to receive training than age groups in the middle; moreover, the oldest cohort got half as many hours of hands-on instruction as any other segment of the work force. The ratio of informal training to formal training for workers over 55 exceeds that for younger ones (Butler et al., 1999: 203–5; Goldberg, 2000: 164). The cost of training mature workers, according to many corporate managers, simply does not justify the payoff. Insofar as employers feel that retirement should be an aging employee's next career move, prospects for advancement or new assignments diminish, making an older person's departure from the firm all the more inevitable (Kumashiro, 2003: 156).

Employees themselves respond in mixed ways to training. The willingness to enroll in job-related classes is directly related to years of prior education according to a 2001 study. Those with at least some college education signed up for courses in business technology more frequently than those with high-school educations. More than half of those who took computer courses did so on their own initiative, paying for classes themselves. That said, the cost of self-education was a barrier for 43 percent of the aged cohort (Morrow et al., 2001: 73). Older workers are also deterred by the negative signals they receive from their managers. They see little point in obtaining new skills absent an assurance that there is a chance for promotion at the end of the training. Some are anxious about returning to the classroom. Older workers are self-conscious about their writing skills and their ability to keep up with younger employees closer to their student days. Older people are sometimes afraid that the experiences gained in the workplace will neither compensate for learning deficiencies nor aid them in learning new skills (Bluestone et al., 1990: 131).

This concatenation of attitudes, policies, and structures pushes older workers into retirement. Nevertheless, in recent decades other factors are causing employers and employees alike to question prevailing structural barriers and ageist assumptions. Population aging is going to force managers of U.S. businesses and industries to make the (re)training of older workers a major priority (Mital, 2003). In less than a decade, half the American labor force will be over 45. A projected shortage of younger workers will put a premium on retaining men and women with experience and loyalty who are healthier and better educated than previous older cohorts. Global aging raises the stakes: unless this country wishes to increase the extent to which it outsources the manufacturing of basic goods and the delivery of information technologies to other countries, it will have to improve the technological competencies of its own human-resource pool (Goldberg, 2000: xiv, 11; Morrow-Howell et al., 2001: 188; Lorenz, 2005). Thus, increasing numbers of U.S. corporations understand the value of upgrading the skills of workers over 45 to remain competitive locally and globally.

Many decision makers in U.S. firms are recognizing the advantages of increasing the work-life potential and assets of older workers (typically defined as those over 40). For the economy to grow, workers must have the skills to be productive in meaningful activities. To make this happen, the United States must invest in training designed to meet the real needs of a changing labor market. Besides offering classes in information technology, it is necessary to upgrade the basic literacy skills of both old (and young) workers.

Meeting the education needs of mature workers will be a priority in an aging workforce. For example, we should increase the scope and financing of federal employment and training programs such as the Job Training Partnership Act (JTPA). This program currently serves a small fraction of men between the ages of 55 and 64 compared to those between 22 and 44—though it does reach a significant percentage of displaced, unemployed homemakers between 45 and 54 (Bluestone et al., 1990: 137–39; Bass et al., 2003: 225). A major structural challenge, as I discuss in the next chapter, is that there is currently a disconnect between what colleges and universities offer through their adult education programs and the vocational and technological skills that older workers need to perform their jobs well. We should initiate more partnerships between institutions of higher education and JTPA, which currently underwrites greater training under the aegis of private industry than through institutions of higher learning.

Similarly, few older workers take advantage of programs such as the Senior Community Service Employment Program, which provides 61,000 subsidized jobs authorized under the Older Americans Act. Working with AARP, Green Thumb, and the National Council on the Aging, this initiative has enabled 100,000 older people to provide services to their communities. Yet Congress has not earmarked funds for educational initiatives or serious retraining under this program (Bass et al., 1993: 225; CFDA, 2002). The Senior Community Service Employment Program's mandate could be adapted to teach skills that could be transferred from the voluntary sector to the marketplace. At present other institutions partially fill the learning gap.

Unions are moving beyond their slogan of the 1940s—"Too Old to Work, Too Young to Die." Besides negotiating better pensions for blue- and white-collar workers in heavy industry, some unions now provide limited retraining opportunities. At times the learning experiences occur in union halls; sometimes they take place in nearby community colleges. Unions also offer pre-retirement counseling as well as venues to engage in social, political, and organizational activities (Bluestone et al., 1990: 71–73). But like most institutions, they tend to stick to doing what they know best how to deliver within the purview of activities under their own control.

Campus-based senior education programs have laid the foundation for (re)training programs. Initiatives in higher education will be more fully discussed in the next chapter, but it is important to note here that more can be done to build on partnerships with corporations in implementing programs for mature workers. Most of the training is indirect: those over the age of 30 constitute a significant proportion of those who enroll in community college courses. Significantly, educators rely on new technologies to deliver their subject matter—often using the very equipment that older workers use on their jobs. Faculty in many private colleges and public universities offer distance-education courses via television or video. Typically senior citizens are given discounts or pay no tuition for such classes. A few colleges and universities make the needs and desires of older students a priority. For example, a fifth of the student body of Saddleback College in California consists of retirees in its Emeritus Institute, and Ekerdt College in Florida attracts many elderly adults (Bass et al., 1993: 224).

Two alternatives in educating older Americans are also worth mentioning. On the one hand, there are freestanding programs that offer classes on campuses. Elderhostel is a good example. Founded in 1975, Elderhostel is a nonprofit institution that now offers roughly 10,000 programs in ninety countries to 200,000 men and women over 55. Primarily concerned with offering intellectually challenging experiences in learning, Elderhostel has not included in its mission a role in helping businesses and firms to upgrade workers' skills (Elderhostel, 2004). On the other hand, the University of Phoenix, founded in 1976, does appeal to consumers who want to improve their technological competencies. The university became the first accredited institution of higher learning to offer degree programs over the Internet. Its faculty work closely with companies in developing curricula. With more than 17,000 instructors and 128 campuses worldwide, it claims that 171,000 working people have earned degrees (University of Phoenix, 2004).

For the present, U.S. companies are likely to adapt to remain competitive here and abroad. Upgrading the skills of older workers is a way to improve the quality of the labor force. "Businesses, in re-examining their assumptions about lifetime employment, must also be willing to make some investments in future training," argues Frank Doyle. "It clearly is a critical need for the mid-career work force caught in the transition from the era of 'career employment with one firm' to the era of 'an employment career with several firms.' Lifetime learning is going to be the lubricant for that transition to new employment" (Bluestone, 1990: 292; see also Miller and Cook-Greuter, 2000).

Following the lead of General Motors and McDonald's, there are more than 2,200 in-house corporate "universities" today. Companies reach more older adults than do colleges and universities. Employers in 2003 spent $57 billion on their "learning-by-doing" training programs, largely aimed at mature workers. The Oracle Corporation, for example, employs 1,200 instructors and has underwritten partnerships with a hundred universities at a cost of $50 million. When GTE had to downsize, it offered training courses to those with graduate degrees, calculating that these workers would thereby be appropriately qualified to return to their former positions when the company got new contracts and expanded. Corporations have developed case-based problem-solving curricula similar to ones used by law, medical, and business schools for more than a century (Konrad, 2001; case examples from Goldberg, 2000: 166, 168–69).

Companies report that it is cheaper to retrain employees of any age than to pay severance packages and recruiting costs, not to mention socializing new employees to the firm. Merck and Company claims that training a replacement costs 150 percent of that recruit's starting salary, once expenses such as the production lost due to vacancies and interviewing are factored in. The higher the level of skills sought, the higher the price. Significantly, experiences at Philips Lighting, a high-tech firm, challenge the assumption that older workers must be taught differently from younger ones. Like elementary school teachers, instructors at Philips Lighting like to keep class size small to improve learning outcomes. The experiences of corporate pacesetters show that continuing education and retraining revitalizes not only workers but corporations as well (Goldberg, 2000: 165, 174).

Training and retraining employees, especially those in the second half of their work careers, is the most important thing the United States can do to ensure a competent, productive labor pool amid population aging. But it is not the only strategy to be deployed. Both the public and the private sectors have introduced other measures designed to entice older workers to remain in the marketplace under conditions that satisfy their needs and desires. For instance, lawmakers have adapted Social Security to give retirees more leeway to work part-time. The architects of Social Security imposed a stringent earnings test on those who opted to continue working while collecting benefits. At first retirees were not permitted to earn more than several thousand dollars a year. Once they reached that ceiling, $1 of every $2 of Social Security benefits that they would have earned was withheld. The logic was clear-cut: if senior citizens chose to retire, then they should forego salaries. For decades critics charged that the ceiling was too low, penalizing older people who wanted to work a little. Modest changes periodically were made in the test. In 2000 President Clinton signed the Senior Citizens Freedom to Work Act. The measure eliminated the earnings test for 800,000 workers who had reached the "normal retirement age" (65 to 67, depending on one's birth date). A modified test still applies for those who retired below the normal retirement age to preserve the value of long-term benefits for the very old, especially aged widows (Center for Retirement Research, 2002). Many economists anticipated that the act would have "some, but a relatively modest, effect on overall work activity" (Greenstein, 2000). Still, it was an important symbolic gesture, signaling a desire to eliminate barriers to work in later years under Social Security.

Changing Social Security's earnings test and retraining mature workers are two institutional mechanisms for retaining the older segment of the labor market. Pragmatic companies employ other options. Phased retirement, for instance, was designed decades ago to ease the transition of older workers out of the labor force while affording companies time to train their replacements. What follows are a few recent policies, some borrowed from Japan and western Europe, that have been successful in extending work careers in innovative ways. They may become more widespread in industries and businesses in the United States (Goldberg, 2000: 152–60, 173, 183–85; Bluestone et al., 1990: 101, 143, 403–5; Visser and Beatty, 2003: 8; O. Mitchell, 1993: 138–39; Kumashiro, 2003).

Offering Flexible Time on the Job

Part-time Permanent Work, enabling older workers to be on the job a few days a week or a few hours each day, though they no longer put in forty hours a week.

Temporary or Seasonal Work, which is not expected to last beyond the holidays or a crunch period when employers require extra help.

On-Call Work, also temporary in nature, but less predictable in timing and duration. It affords institutions back-up support from a cadre of experienced workers.

Creative Work Arrangements

Job Redesign is an approach to "repotting" senior employees. The option should start with workers in their prime. By eliminating stress and monotony, motivation rises. It also plants seeds in the minds of employees and employers alike that job flexibility permits fresh thinking and fresh challenges.

Transferring a worker from one job to another position is analogous to job redesign. Sometimes the reassignment comes with fewer responsibilities, ushering in phased retirement.

Consulting for One's Former Employer. Under this scenario, the worker retires and collects a pension. The pensioner returns to work hoping to regain his or her prior position permanently when the economic climate improves or downsizing is completed. Sometimes consulting takes older workers to assignments abroad.

Consulting for Another Employer is a variation on this theme. Secure in the pension vested with one firm, a mature worker can afford to take a less remunerative position elsewhere if the assignment seems appealing.

Job Sharing, an option crafted with young working mothers in mind, can be adapted so that companies retain valued older workers without incurring the costs that come with seniority rules.

Telecommunicating permits an older retiree to use the Internet at home to collaborate with former colleagues who remain at the job site.

Bridge Employment permits a retiree to serve the company in a disaster or to represent the firm in community service.

Mentoring is a way of tapping senior workers to preserve institutional memories and to prepare younger workers to understand the corporate ethos.

Age-Specific Benefits

Subsidies for job (re)training, especially targeted for older workers whose future value to a firm is recognized.

Health Care is critical in the absence of a universal health insurance plan. Amid skyrocketing costs in medical care, many retirees would gladly trade income for fuller coverage for hospitalization and long-term care than afforded under Medicare or that they can buy from Blue Cross/Blue Shield. Older workers are willing to have their employer defray the cost in paying premiums in lieu of a higher salary in some part-time, seasonal, flexible arrangements. Experts indicate, however, that workers' preferences should be surveyed. Some older workers really want the money; they prefer to cover their own health costs.

Ergonomics. Industrial designers underscore the importance of comfortable furniture and good lighting, especially for those who do desk work. Frequent breaks are especially important to mature workers.

Reimbursement for all expenses (travel, meals) associated with working past the normal retirement age.

U.S. companies have already begun to implement these plans. According to Beverly Goldberg (2000: 150), a survey of more than 2,700 human resources managers revealed that 62 percent hired elderly consultants, nearly half provided training to improve mature workers' skills, and roughly 30 percent gave their workers the option to transfer to jobs with fewer responsibilities and less pay. (Surprisingly, only a fifth provided phased-retirement plans, and only a tenth created alternative career paths for their aging workers.) Well-known companies—ranging from fast-food chains, discount stores, hotels, and food processors to insurance companies—take pride in their policies to benefit older workers (see, for instance, *Business Chronicle,* 2000; DelMonte Foods, 2001). AARP periodically salutes the "Best Employers for Workers over 50." In 2003 AARP praised 27 establishments, including Whirlpool and the Massachusetts Institute of Technology, for their efforts to be more flexible in dealing with seasoned workers and in ensuring that they had acquired the skills to stay on the job. "This is a sure indicator of the growing importance of the older worker to the success of individual companies and, in fact, to the entire economy," declared AARP president Jim Parkel (AARP, 2003a; see also Wells Fargo Elder Services, 2004).

Surveys by AARP, the federal government, and the Travelers Company have demonstrated that a certain subgroup of retirees want to "unretire," that is, to return to the labor force in some capacity (Achenbaum and Morrison, 1993: 112). It is highly unlikely, however, that institutional innovations would suffice to lure a majority of senior citizens back into the labor pool. The labor market is so segmented that some policies will work more effectively in certain sectors (such as white-collar positions and sales) than in others. A significant percentage of octogenarians are too disabled or ill to continue working. Others, tired of working in boring jobs, look forward to enjoying their leisure time. Human resources managers, moreover, do not have to rely solely on mature workers to fill labor shortages. They can use robots and other forms of automation to replace people's jobs. They can design family leave policies and child care facilities that would make it easier for women with young children to stay at work. They can outsource jobs to other countries where wages are far lower (Riker, 1997). But we have come a long way from the Townsendite assumption that all older people are unproductive. Mature workers will become an increasingly important component of the labor force. Demography and the quest for productive workers require companies to adapt their procedures to retain the services and loyalty of seasoned workers.

Marketing to the Mature Consumer

U.S. firms and businesses are not the only institutions that have belatedly discovered the potential value of older Americans. The media and advertisers have for several decades been trying to figure out how to tap the "gold in gray" (Minkler and Estes, 1991: 81). In many ways the story of how businesses have clung to distorted views of elderly people as producers parallels the myopia with which marketers have perceived them as consumers. Ageism is the prime culprit in both instances.

David Wolfe, one of the nation's most astute analysts of "the new customer majority" (that is, adults over 40 who constitute mainstream consumer population), claims that Madison Avenue is "stuck in the 1960s." This is having a devastating effect on "corporate America, including equity markets depressed by anemic profits, and on the national economy. . . . The so-called aging of America (and all other developed nations) is dramatically, if not radically, changing the rules of marketplace engagement" (Wolfe and Snyder, 2003: 9–10, 12). Robert Snyder, who heads J. Walter Thompson's Mature Market Group, agrees: "As researchers have become more sophisticated in their approaches to and understanding of human behavior, one would think that new methods of marketing and creative advertising communications would have evolved over the past 50 years. While strides have been made, when all the bells and whistles are stripped away, the strategies of today's advertisers are similar to those used in the 1950's" (U.S. Senate Special Committee on Aging, 2002: 28).

Television executives at ABC and CBS focus on viewers between the ages of 18 and 49 because the strategy pays off: "The fact is that a smaller, younger audience can generate more advertising dollars, and we rely on ad dollars alone as a source of revenue" (quoted in T. E. Robinson, 1998: 9). When elderly people dominate the viewing audience, networks derive less income per show. Creative directors of new networks also pitch to younger age groups because it is more profitable (CommInfoStudies, 2004: 8).

Studies over the past three decades document that twisted images of age have become less pervasive, but they are still rampant. Older people tended to be marginalized in the 1970s; they played peripheral roles or were absent altogether. Aronoff (1974) and Northcott (1975) independently found that only 1.5 percent to 5 percent of the actors in primetime television programming were elderly. Only 2 percent of all commercials showed any elderly characters (Francher, 1973). Older women were less visible than men—only one out of ten elderly characters was a woman. Sixty percent of the portrayals of these older characters, moreover, were negative—ineffectual, unhappy, or unattractive.

Thirty years later slight progress has been made. Elders starred in popular shows such as *Golden Girls, Murder She Wrote,* and *Matlock.* Instead of cameo appearances, some older actors got supporting roles. Lower-class characters were featured. Yet unless they were well known and esteemed for their portrayal of late life, elderly people remained under-represented in television. A survey of spots on ABC, CBS, NBC, and Fox included only 42 aged figures, compared to 100 youthful characters and 174 who were middle-aged. Of the 42, in only 15 were older persons featured in solo performances; 21 spots allocated minor roles to older persons, and 6 portrayed youth and age together. Older actors outnumbered older actresses, but the gap has declined. Less than 2 percent of the elderly actors were African American or of Hispanic origin (Tupper, 1995).

Cross-national studies reveal a similar pattern. Japan, which has the world's largest percentage of older citizens, has traditionally venerated elders. Yet a comparison of children's programs in Japan and the United States revealed that only 4 percent of the Japanese elders had speaking roles, compared to 9 percent in the United States. Only 2 percent of the Japanese figures were women. Japanese characters remained on the screen for only a third of the time of their American counterparts (Delloff, 1987; for Britain, see Featherstone, 1991). Some experts fear that the invisibility of elders in children's shows may presage strained intergenerational relations in decades ahead.

The relative paucity of older characters on television shows and in commercials is ironic because elderly Americans watch more television for longer periods of time than do younger age groups. "Old people today generally are not appreciated as experienced 'elders' or possessors of special wisdom; they are simply seen as sometimes remaining competent enough to be included in the unitary role category of 'active citizen,'" observes Meyrowitz (1985: 153) in critiquing the place of elderly Americans in the media. "Old people are respected to the extent that they can behave like young people, that is, to the extent that they remain capable of working, enjoying sex, exercising, and taking care of themselves." As is the case in the labor force, ignoring the elderly cohort sends a message. When only young people are shown driving new, sporty cars, TV viewers presume that older people do not buy or drive luxury cars. Shots of crowds in fast-food restaurants that do not include gray hairs and bald heads leave the impression that older people do not frequent such businesses.

Worse, when older people are portrayed in the media and in advertising, they are still too often shown in unflattering ways. Pharmaceutical advertising is an exception to this generalization: 85 percent of the advertisements in the broad media targeted at senior citizens feature health matters such as medicine, vitamins, and health insurance (U.S. Senate Special Committee on Aging, 2003: 30; T. E. Robinson, 1998: 66). Television advertisements tend to be more stereotypic toward older people than magazines or newspapers in messages aimed at younger populations. Nearly a third of all advertisements targeted to the older market on television are negative, far greater than found in magazines and newspapers. Only in advertisements directed to all consumers is ageism reduced; researchers attribute the decline to the fact that elderly people are part of the scene but do not dominate it (T. E. Robinson, 1998: 63). Not only do negative images shape younger people's impressions of what it means to grow older, but elderly people themselves react poorly to inaccurate portrayals: a slim majority claim that they would stop using a product that was presented in the media in a way that denigrated aged persons (ibid.: 35).

Nor are popular, seasoned veterans of the media secure in their jobs. In 2002, ABC began negotiating with late-night comic host David Letterman to take over the spot held by prize-winning reporter Ted Koppel on *Nightline*. Letterman apparently had "long been unhappy with CBS's older prime time audience." The average age of his audience was 46; Koppel's average viewer was 52. That difference translated into a thirty-second ad rate of $40,000 for Letterman compared to $30,000 for Koppel—despite the fact that *Nightline* had a 10 percent greater audience. On Madison Avenue, "a program can win its ratings' war but still be considered a loser because its audience is older. It will make less money" (U.S. Senate, Special Committee on Aging, 2003: 66; Wolfe, 2003: 11). Executives at National Public Radio apparently did not care that the host of its *Morning Edition* had doubled its audience over the past decade when it decided to force out its host, Bob Edwards, who had been the program's "iconic figure" since its inception in 1979. NPR declared that "it's part of a natural evolution" that "had to do with the changing needs of our listeners. . . . It was a programming decision about the right sound" (CNN.com, 2004; Washingtonpost.com, 2004). Both companies gave priority to young, not old, viewers.

The structural and cultural ageism found in the media and marketing arises from several causes. Negative images of late life are deeply rooted in Western culture. Once there were relatively few older people in society, and those who survived past fifty generally were poor and/or afflicted with some sort of ailment. Generation after generation has coined derogatory terms to disesteem the value of age: Americans derided one who did not keep up with the times as a "fogy" (1830); a "geezer" was the epithet for someone who acted peculiarly; and around the turn of the century, a "fuddy duddy" was just too fastidious. Sometimes positive terms such as "gaffer" acquired negative connotations (Fischer, 1977; Achenbaum, 1978b). In the 1950s, Americans referred to their elders as "dinosaurs" and "blue-hairs." Lately, words such as "gerry" and "trog" have entered the lexicon (Nunberg, 2004). Even flippant terms such as "p"s or "rents" to refer to parents have the effect of belittling maturity in a culture of youth.

It is little wonder that Generation X and its successor, with money to burn, appeal to marketers. "Advertisers pay a premium for young adults because, with their expanding families and recent entry into the grown-up marketplace, they are supposed to spend the most on packaged goods and services that advertise on television" (Butler et al., 1999: 232). According to ACNielsen, advertisers spend $23.54 per thousand adults aged 18 to 34, compared to $9.57 for those over 34. Nonetheless, innovative marketers are beginning to acknowledge that concentrating on a 15-year age span is limiting.

Advertising executives and media experts are grappling with another set of hard data that potentially translates into serious revenues. Older men and women not only are the heaviest users of television but also are the most numerous and loyal subscribers to newspapers and magazines. (They attend movies less frequently than younger and middle-aged Americans.) Far from being passive viewers, older people are estimated to represent 40 percent of the consumer demand in the country. Furthermore, this age group actually pays attention to the commercials and the sales. More than three-fifths of all senior citizens claim that commercials are "often or always helpful" in determining what purchases to make (T. E. Robinson, 1998: 6).

Furthermore, those in the second half of life have the economic wherewithal to satisfy their needs and desires. Men and women over 50 hold half the nation's credit cards. According to the U.S. Administration on Aging, the median net worth of a household headed by someone between the ages of 55 and 64 was $145,000; between 65 and 74, $190,000; and those over 75, $132,900 (CommInfoStudies, 2004). Responding to new demographic and economic realities, companies such as Toyota, Bud Light, Coca-Cola, and McDonald's are starting to use older actors in their advertisements. The fashion industry is designing clothes for working women between the ages of 55 and 64. Travel companies lure well-off folk ("woofies"). Dockers, L. L. Bean, and other manufacturers of leisure wear are redesigning sizes to accommodate their customers' widening waistlines (T. E. Robinson, 1998: 11).

Finally, globalization negates any justification for depicting the elderly population as homogeneous. As we have already seen, each cohort of the U.S. population is more ethnically diverse than the older one above it. When we export goods to Europe, China, India, and South America, commercials and advertisements must illustrate our diversity to the world. And therein lies a structural disconnect. How should advertisers cultivate an international market as it appeals to U.S. customers?

"The mature market is full of contradictions," the *Wall Street Journal* opined more than fifteen years ago (Butler et al., 1999: 225). No single factor predicts how older people will respond to inducements to buy items regularly. Mature consumers do not like high-pressure tactics, but they enjoy shopping, especially for well-known products. Some older people exercise by walking in shopping malls, often purchasing something they see in a store window. For them, going to the mall is recreational. Other data present a different type of older consumer: it describes a subset reluctant to try new outlets, one not very confident in selecting items to buy. Some older people, adept on the Internet, bid on eBay and select purchases through catalogs and magazines; other consumers want to examine the product, especially if it is expensive, before they make a purchase (Lumpkin et al., 1989: 177).

Thus far, marketers have generally opted for three strategies in appealing to mature consumers. One tack focuses on the product itself, then reaches out to the segment they wish to capture (Morgan and Levy,

2002: 2). Advertisers "cream" the affluent segment of the mature market, enticing them with luxury cruises to exotic places or clothes and cosmetics that flatter their appearance. Home builders perceive men and women over 55 to be their fastest-growing market. Their research reveals divergent needs and preferences. One subset is likely to relocate to the Sunbelt; another wants to downsize because they are finished raising their children. Some modernize their existing residence by remodeling. Still others plan for a caregiver moving in, when necessary, to help with a bedridden or severely incapacitated owner. Builders prepare special manuals for their sales force to explain the intricacies of selling, buying, and renovating in clear, simple terms. Those who interact with mature clients avoid stereotypic words such as *ambulate* or *challenged,* opting instead to extol the *comfortability* and *individual choices* at stake (Tuccillo et al., 1995; Kelly, 2003).

Marketers are attempting to create a niche within the elderly population while remaining close to the mainstream preferences of consumers of all ages. The strategy is not always consistent. Advertisers may use middle-aged or older women as models in selling beauty products, but their copy promises that the customer will "feel" and "look" younger. The promise of youth is not mentioned in media presentations in which older women sell laxatives, dental fixtures, or remedies for aches and pains (T. E. Robinson, 1998: 10; Ives, 2004).

A second group of market researchers have analyzed psychological attitudes and behavioral measures, demographic data, and social indicators to segment the mature market so as to identify a range of products that might appeal to particular subsets. One of the pioneers in this area was Rena Bartos, who divided people over 50 into six groups based on how they used their time and adjusted to financial and health changes during the second half of life. Bartos recommended that marketers focus on "active affluents," "active retireds," and "homemakers," who made up 75 percent of the population. She ignored "the disadvantaged," those who are in poor health, and "others" (Moschis, 1996: 47). Subsequent work has shown that age-based bracketing and cohort analyses are too general because of the diversity of income and needs within the boundaries of the group identified. Lifestyles are a component of any profile, but they do not provide empirical evidence that social status drives consumption patterns. Nor does it work to aim products at people in a particular geographic area (Morgan and Levy, 2002: 31, 33).

Perhaps the most ambitious endeavor in this genre is George Moschis's *Gerontographics,* "an attempt to gain insight into human behavior in late life by recognizing the multifaceted aspects of the aging process, and [by considering] consumer behavior to be a manifestation of these multidimensional processes and circumstances" (1996: 54). Moschis used 136 redundant measures because he felt that no smaller set of factors sufficed. He dissected similarities and differences in values and health as well as behavioral and social connectedness among diverse subsets of the older population. Based on his elaborate typology, Moschis recommended market strategies for specific items. For instance, he said that "healthy indulgers" looked for sales on foods that were nutritional and aromatic. "Ailing outgoers" also wanted rebates, but they were more interested in products that were easy to use with clear labels and instructions (ibid.: 128). Critics praised the way Moschis incorporated previous studies into his model but wondered whether a typology that was so industry-specific yet that acknowledged marked variations within subgroup consumption patterns was a truly effective approach.

A third strategy for reaching the mature market focuses on values that "cut across all age groups" (U.S. Senate Special Committee on Aging, 2003: 25). Avowedly postmodern in orientation, this tack presumes that the diversity of consumption patterns in late life arise from the proliferation of "contingent life strategies" that emerge over individuated life courses. Senior citizens define for themselves their own meaningful identities and appropriate body images. *Maturity* is the keyword in this approach, for it affirms the ripening that comes with advancing years. It also masks physical and mental decline as well as the psychological and social disconnectedness evident among some older persons. Accentuating the positive, active features of vital aging, values-oriented marketers declare: "Don't call 'Em Old, Call 'Em Consumers" (S. Katz, 1999: 8–9; Katz and Marshall, 2003: 5).

David Wolfe coined the phrase "Ageless Marketing" to describe this third strategy for reaching the hearts and minds of mature consumers. His Center for Ageless Marketing builds on recent research on how brains detect and react to information, consciously forming distinctive thoughts and decisions. "Through the miracle of neuroimaging, brain researchers can now eavesdrop on the goings on between a person's ears as thoughts are being formed and decisions made" (Center for Ageless Marketing, 2003: xi). Wolfe then melds this path-breaking scientific tool with lessons from developmental psychology to form a paradigmatic lens for understanding the senior market: "At age 23, Jamie Lee Curtis would not have imagined showing off her love handles in a popular magazine. But a 43-year-old Jamie is not just a 20-year-older version of her 23-year-old self. She is in many ways a different person. However, the person she is today evolved along a somewhat predictable path" (Wolfe, 2003: 19, 37, 82; see also Walker, 2005). Curtis, like many of the rest of us, learned to satisfy basic needs and, with time and experience, attain a state of self-actualization that determines how we feel, how we see ourselves, and how we want to continue to grow.

Symptomatic of the ageless market is the unprecedented effort to address sexual dysfunctions in later years. Researchers such as Robert Butler and Myrna Lewis (1976), among others, provided empirical evidence that "sex after sixty" was not an oxymoron. Older people, claimed Butler and Lewis, desired intimacy as much as younger persons; they were capable of satisfying their desires, often in ways more sensual than they had enjoyed earlier in their lives. Recently, biomedical scientists and psychologists encouraged women who felt that they may be experiencing female sexual arousal disorder to discuss the malady with their physicians to seek relief. Urometrics created a Web site to facilitate dialog and successfully targeted Eros Therapy for older women (Katz and Marshall, 2003: 10–12). Hormone-replacement therapies found a lucrative market among aging and menopausal women. Other sex-enhancing devices and techniques became available. That companies began to invest in such pharmaceutical interventions and mechanical treatments attests to their newfound conviction that sexual satisfaction is important to women as they age—and potentially profitable to them.

Men's sexual difficulties, notably erectile dysfunction, were also openly discussed. Viagra, a little blue pill created by Pfizer to remedy what urologists considered an organic problem, was advertised in all the media, including Super Bowl commercials (the most costly advertising slot in the United States). Pfizer chose Robert Dole, the 1996 Republican presidential candidate who had experienced impotence after prostate surgery five years earlier, to attest to the restorative powers of Viagra (Associated Press, 1998). Dole, then a 75-year-old U.S. senator, gave the product the credibility it needed. Pfizer gradually recognized that Viagra could reach a market even wider than older men. Young couples in their 30s and 40s embracing each other started to replace images of gray-haired couples dancing. "The pill becomes one more tool in the project of constructing the sexually functional male body—with both its maleness and its functionality defined by penile erectility—as an ageless body, a project which now must begin earlier and earlier in the life course" (Marshall and Katz, 2002: 61).

Ageless marketing, by conjoining consumer behavior and life-course studies, emphasizes the salience of lifelong values and continuities in lifestyle preferences. In so doing, it serves to integrate young and old consumer populations. The strategy parallels modifications in human-resource policies that afford mature workers more opportunities to spend their retirement in productive, constructive, satisfying ways. Yet by accentuating the positive features of growing older, ageless marketing may unwittingly bolster the agenda of the anti-aging faction of gerontology, which is convinced that science will someday extend life expectancy considerably by eliminating the deleterious features of old age (S. Katz, 1999: 3, 12).

Ironically, ageless marketing, which originally focused on a burgeoning segment of the population, might render invisible those elders whose wrinkles, low income, and ethnic diversity do not fit the advertisers' portrayal of successful aging. If so, then ageless marketing may itself represent a new manifestation of ageism in a population that is rapidly aging. But it is too early to tell. "Gerontology should welcome further scholarship on consumers, commodities, and consumption as a way to understand how this activity shapes and tugs the contemporary idea of age" (Ekerdt, 2004b: S57).

(Re)Creating Networks for Lifelong Learning and Sharing Talents } 3

"We have gone far beyond the ancient adage, 'If youth only knew, and age only could,'" declared 70-year-old philosopher and educator John Dewey (1939: xxv). "For there is now no socially organized means by which the aged have (or at least are supposed to have) even the *knowledge* which is relevant to the conditions of social life, much less the opportunity of applying it." Dewey had devoted his career to building institutions in which children, youth, and middle-aged people could acquire those skills and perspectives necessary to enable them to grapple with various societal problems inherent in democracies. Now, as he wrote an introduction to the first multidisciplinary U.S. gerontology handbook, *Problems of Ageing* (Cowdry, 1939), he pondered why the nation tolerated institutional barriers diminishing older people's fuller engagement in society.

The "acquisition of skills, possession of knowledge, attainment of culture are not ends: they are marks of growth and means to its continuing," Dewey had written two years earlier in *Reconstruction in Philosophy.* "Government, business, art, religion, all social institutions have a meaning," he declared. "That purpose is to set free and to develop the capacities of human individuals without respect to race, sex, class or economic status" (1937: 185–86). Insofar as education afforded a scientifically grounded lifelong process toward maturation, individuals, regardless of age, should learn how to contribute to the well-being of the commonweal. Yet old people, in Dewey's opinion, lacked the training and institutional support to participate in this noble service.

As a first step to remedying the situation, Dewey recommended "study to ascertain and develop the kind of activities in which the older part of the population can engage with satisfaction to themselves and value to the community. . . . With the prospect of over a third of the total population above fifty years in age, it is a pressing problem" (Dewey, 1939: xxiv). Consistent with his theories of human development, Dewey hoped that systematic research into adult intelligence would undercut the prevailing belief among experts and citizens alike that "old dogs could not learn new tricks." No one doubted that cognitive capacities declined over the life course; the issue was how severe the decrements were. George Beard asserted in *American Nervousness* (1881: 250) that "the querulousness of age, the irritability, the avarice are partly of habit and partly of organic and functional changes in the brain." In *Principles of Psychology* (1890: II, 1910), William James argued that people found it harder to assimilate new ideas with advancing years: "Old-fogyism . . . is the inevitable terminus to which life sweeps us on." James's use of "fogy" was consistent with its definition in the 1880 edition of Webster's *American Dictionary* as "a dull old fellow, a person behind the times, overconservative, or slow." With few exceptions "amid the general wreck of bodily and cerebral powers," claimed W. A. Newland Dorland in *The Age of Mental Virility* (1908: 70), the mental capabilities of persons over 60 were impaired.

During the first third of the twentieth century, a few scholars and popular writers challenged the assumption that older people were doomed to become "geezers." In *Senescence* (1922: 405–7), psychologist G. Stanley Hall hypothesized that "intelligent and well-conserved senectitude has very important social and anthropological functions in the world." Eduard C. Lindeman, a friend and colleague of John Dewey, stated in *The Meaning of Adult Education* (1926) that education in later life had nonvocational aims. Applying a lifetime of experiences guided learners more as they confronted life's uncertain voyage than mastering a prescribed curriculum (Infed, 2004). Yet even the revisionists admitted limits to how much intellect could be maintained with advancing years. While celebrating that *Life Begins at Forty,* Walter Pitkin warned his readers that "your level of best performance after forty will probably be at least one step below that on which you succeeded before forty" (1932:

48). And *Adult Learning,* considered the definitive study at the time, conceded that "the degenerative effect of age . . . at about fifty-five the net
result of changes in general energy, interest in one's work, and ability to
improve is a regression in achievement" (Thorndike et al., 1928: 131).
If the intellectual curve fell dramatically in the fifth decade, there seemed
to be little point in providing learning opportunities to those over 60.

Dewey conceded as much: "I do not think it is too much to say that
this whole field [of adult education, especially for elderly persons] is a
practical blank at the present time. There are here and there individuals
who have managed to work out a solution, but as far as I can see, such
cases are a matter of combination of a fortunate personal temperament
and lucky surroundings" (1939: xxiv). Dewey may have had in mind the
pioneering work of Dr. Lillien J. Martin, a retired head of Stanford University's Department of Psychology. Beginning with *Salvaging Old Age*
(1930), Martin described the philosophy and techniques that she used
in aiding elders who no longer desired to live life fully. The aim of her
Old Age Counseling Center in San Francisco, opened in 1929, was "the
permanent development and growth of every client, measured in terms
of his useful participation in the life in the community in which he finds
himself, for increased happiness and efficiency" (Martin, 1944: 72). Dr.
William McKeever, another retired educator, opened a "school for mat-
urates" in Oklahoma City in the 1930s. These creative ventures stressed
the importance of offering adult learners access to education. Because
these are not the only prototypes for current educational programs for
older Americans, it is worth reviewing the state of adult education before
World War II.

Adult Education in the United States, from Benjamin Franklin to John Dewey

Children and youth always have been the primary beneficiaries of
the nation's educational structure (Cremin, 1970–88). The Boston Latin
School (1635) was the first town-supported school in the British colonies;
three years later the Dutch Reformed Church established a religious-
based school in New Amsterdam. Protestant denominations founded
nine colleges between 1636 and 1769; a few missionaries sought to teach
Native Americans, African Americans, and poor whites to read and
write. After the founding of the Republic, the federal government and

various states supported private educational efforts. The Northwest Ordinance of 1787 required frontier townships to set aside land for schools. States established boards of education in the 1830s and 1840s that set minimum standards for school attendance. While boys received preferential treatment in elementary and secondary schools, some reformers gave priority to the instruction of young ladies: Horace Mann established "normal schools" to train school teachers in Massachusetts in 1839; "seminaries" were precedents for women's colleges established after the Civil War.

Educators filled in other gaps as the system evolved. The Freedman's Bureau, which established nearly 3,000 schools before curtailing its academic division in 1870, contributed to the growth of Howard University, Tuskegee Institute, and Spelman College. States mandated stringent compulsory attendance and child labor laws so that schools could "Americanize" new waves of immigrants. The first Manual Training School for boys (1879) became the basis for vocational tracks in high schools around the turn of the century. Jane Addams's Hull House (1889) inspired the building of a hundred settlement houses to teach mothers domestic skills and their children vocational training along with lessons in the responsibilities of citizenship.

The purpose, size, and scope of institutions of higher education changed during the second half of the nineteenth century. The Morrill Act (1862) gave states land to sell so that legislatures would create colleges offering advanced instruction in "applied" studies. Elite colleges expected their faculty to do specialized research while teaching undergraduates in their disciplines. Progressive universities added professional training in medicine, law, and business to their mission. Meanwhile, innovators such as John Dewey and G. Stanley Hall, armed with new ways to measure intelligence and personalities, transformed ideas about the proper environment for teaching skills to children and youth. High school enrollments grew 650 percent between 1900 and 1930 alone.

By the onset of the Great Depression, a mixture of public and private initiatives at the federal, state, and local levels had created a tripartite division of educational sectors—primary and secondary schools and places of higher learning. Networks were more bureaucratic than they were two centuries earlier, and educators and taxpayers debated different issues than the colonists had. Nonetheless, future accretions would be grafted onto the "modern" infrastructure. Concurrently, an ancillary system was being developed to address the needs of adult learners. Indeed, the origins of continuing education, like the primary school and college, date back to pre-Revolutionary times.

Benjamin Franklin was the Father of Adult Education in this country. He convinced a dozen friends in 1727 to form the Junto, "a school of good manners and good works" (Morgan, 1992: 43). The Junto met weekly to discuss what Franklin in his *Autobiography* described as "Morals, Politics, or Natural Philosophy," to promote participants' prosperity, and to work for the benefit of others. Junto members became the nucleus of the august American Philosophical Society (1743). Concerned from the outset with the study of "useful sciences," the Society remains a center for scholars and scientists who aspire "to multiply the conveniences and pleasures of life" (Martin et al., 2000: 86). Improving working men's minds was another of Franklin's abiding concerns. With the Junto's support he worked to charter the first public library in the British colonies, to which adults could subscribe through a system of fees and fines. Between 1733 and 1758 Franklin also published *Poor Richard's Almanac,* which entertained ordinary readers with aphorisms and practical information.

During the nineteenth century several other significant vehicles for adults to improve themselves emerged. Craft entrepreneurs established mechanics institutes for the urban working class. Based on models in London and Glasgow, the institutes focused on contemporary U.S. political controversies as well as on the dissemination of ideas about commerce, manufacturing, and agriculture (Wilentz, 1984: 150–51). In 1826 Josiah Holbrook launched the Lyceum movement in the United States "to apply the sciences and the various branches of education to the domestic and useful arts, and to all the common purposes of life" (Bode, 1956: 12). Holbrook wanted, among other things, to improve the level of discourse beyond the frivolous exchange of words, to improve public schools, to compile town maps and histories, and to conduct geological and agricultural surveys. By the 1840s, community-based curricula gave way to platform lectures: distinguished figures such as Ralph Waldo Emerson and Dr. Oliver Wendell Holmes were paid $12 to $20 to speak (ibid.: 24–25, 190).

The first Chautauqua Assembly was held in 1874 as a summer camp for Sunday school teachers. Mixing recreation and education, the founders envisioned a lifelong learning center for all ages and educational levels. Campers took classes in religion, music, and art; some signed up for correspondence courses. Offshoots were established by 1886 from Maine to Florida, California to Oregon (Porter, 2004). At the height of the movement, speakers on the Chautauqua circuit journeyed to nearly 10,000 communities each season. (The Ku Klux Klan emulated the program with its own Klan Tauqua.)

Women's clubs played an important role in expanding American adult education. According to the U.S. Department of Labor, there were more than 1,200 such clubs around the turn of the twentieth century. Convinced that women lacked "intellectual training in thoroughness and accuracy" (Kett, 1994: 153), club members embarked on a course of study comparable to that available to men—with an important difference. Men had vocational goals in mind when they joined self-improvement groups. Women of a certain age hoped to broaden their intellectual horizons (Adams, 1944: 138–39). Thus, whereas the summer institutes held at Woods Hole were designed for male scientific researchers, women largely underwrote the Concord Summer School of Philosophy and Felix Adler's Ethical Culture movement, where the likes of John Dewey and Josiah Royce offered their perspectives on recent trends in ethical philosophy (Kett, 1994: 167).

Although other institutions contributed to the adult education movement in the 1900s, few gave high priority to adult learners as they adapted to a new urban-industrial order. The number of libraries in communities with populations over 1,000, for instance, grew from 971 in 1896 to 2,465 in 1925, more than half built by Andrew Carnegie (Learned, 1924: 83). Even so, roughly 37 percent of the American population had no access to library services. Only large urban facilities could supply the scientific and technical material that would justify their being called "the people's university" (Adams, 1944: 223). Furthermore, libraries' purpose changed, becoming increasingly tied to the public school system. They extended borrowing privileges to girls and boys under 10 because "the library's first role, obviously, is to the child" (quoted in Kett, 1994: 219; Learned, 1924: 6). In this context, enriching the minds of older learners did not rank high in the aims of public libraries.

A few educational institutions took steps to reach out to older learners. Innovators noted the considerable success Cambridge and Oxford had in the 1870s and 1880s in drawing mature students to classes taught by extension lecturers. The University of Chicago, whose first president had ties to the Chautauqua movement, inaugurated correspondence courses in the United States in 1892. Shortly thereafter the University of Wisconsin opened an extension center in Milwaukee; the University of Michigan followed suit with one in Detroit. These centers floundered, however, because they could not provide the physical ambiance and intellectual vitality to be found in Madison or Ann Arbor. The success of proprietary correspondence schools depended on how well they solicited potential subscribers to learn through the mail how to become osteopaths, detectives, and missionaries (Kett, 1994: 182, 284, 301; Adams, 1944: 261–62).

Spurred by the Hatch Act (1887), Penn State, among other universities, dispatched lecturers to agricultural areas, but only 4,000 students were enrolled in agricultural extension classes a decade later. Colleges started summer schools so women could obtain teacher certification. Joliet, Illinois, created the nation's first junior college in 1902 to offer inexpensive courses beyond high school for young people. So perhaps it is not surprising that the American Society for the Extension of University Teaching (1893), which aimed to put "new and worthy objects of thought into the lives of people who have been content to live in intellectual sloth and barrenness" (quoted in Kett, 1994: 142), shrunk within a few years, confining activities to the Philadelphia area. In an era that put a premium on efficiency and professional advancement, adult education programs had to be pragmatic in scope to succeed. Learning for its own sake was no longer sustainable either for undergraduates or mature students (ibid.: 187).

To ensure training opportunities appropriate for their needs, corporations and labor unions designed educational programs for adult workers. In 1884, for example, the president of the National Cash Register Company (NCR) inaugurated a program to teach clerks how to sell his product. When sales increased as a result of the venture, the company started separate schools for repairmen and persons who wanted to work in butcher shops, groceries, and drug stores. Sugar companies emulated NCR, as did institutes of banking (which alone enrolled 40,000 students) and iron and steel concerns. Bell Telephone arranged for professors at the University of Pennsylvania to offer a humanities course to rising executives (Kett, 1994: 240, 438; Adams, 1944: 168–69). The newly formed Rotary International offered its members weekly speakers who analyzed national and global affairs as well as concerns of local interest.

Rotary also engaged in vocational education, stressing the importance of ethical behavior in business. Although trade unions were primarily interested in bread-and-butter issues, some were attuned to new trends in adult education. The first resident labor college was launched in Arkansas in 1900. The National Women's Trade Union League established a school for women organizers in 1913. The American Federation of Labor adopted a plan to promote workers' education six years later (Adams, 1944: 205).

The contributions of three other institutions are worth noting. Wealthy collectors donated or bought works of art, scientific instruments, and other cultural objects to be displayed in urban museums, many built in the last quarter of the nineteenth century. Museums became places where people of all ages could view artifacts and masterpieces from other times and places, although curators rarely organized exhibits to enhance viewers' education. More instrumental in its approach was the radio. In addition to airing programs for various ethnic groups, radio further segmented its audience with programs such as "Labor News Flashes," "Musical Potpourri," and "Invitation to Learning," all designed to make high culture palatable to listeners' tastes (Cohen, 1990: 136; Kett, 1994: 376). Finally, philanthropies had a role in developing adult education. The Carnegie Corporation, chartered "to promote the advancement and diffusion of knowledge and understanding among the people of the United States," supported the publication of Edward Thorndike's *Adult Learning* (1928). Eight years later, under the aegis of the American Association for Adult Education, it underwrote twenty-seven "Studies in the Social Significance of Adult Education," in titles such as *Everyman's Drama, Educating for Health, The Church and Adult Education,* and *Education for Social Understanding* (Stubblefield, 1988: 28; Adams, 1944: 354–55).

As it had done in inviting Abraham Flexner, a layperson, to survey medical education at the beginning of the century, the Carnegie Corporation asked James Truslow Adams, editor of the six-volume *Dictionary of American History,* to critique the state of adult education in the United States. In *Frontiers of American Culture* (1944: 128), Adams referred repeatedly to "the adult education jumble." Historian Joseph Kett, writing fifty years later, came to the same conclusion: "By the eve of World War II, adult education had achieved a status at once vast and marginal . . . it became exclusively what it long had been in part, a minor bureaucracy within state and local education departments, university extension divisions, and collegiate schools of education" (Kett, 1994: 401).

Significantly, none of the manifold adult education initiatives viewed older people as their chief stakeholders. No wonder John Dewey considered the field "a practical blank." Adult education was a marginal enterprise; few invested in the old-age market. The situation would not change until educators and older people themselves were convinced that intellectual growth was possible in later years. That is why Dewey recommended that researchers study learning curves more systematically.

Beyond "Adult Learning": Institutional Responses to Andragogy

New perspectives on the cognitive capabilities of older Americans were slow to emerge, but the cumulative effect of psychological, social-scientific, and biomedical research during the twentieth century has been to undermine stereotypic "old-fogyism." The first cohort of investigators took their cues from John Dewey and Eduard Lindeman, among others. These progressive, pragmatic educators expounded a philosophy of education that emphasized the value of older learners' experiences in dealing with the here and now in contrast to training younger students for future eventualities (Werner, 2000: 2; Martin and deGruchy, 1930). After World War II, a new generation of gerontologists demonstrated that older people were capable of learning and performing under suitable conditions. Three examples will suffice. James Birren (1955) made his reputation by demonstrating that the functioning of the nervous system changed with age, slowing reaction times to perceptual cues. His findings were corroborated by A. T. Welford's *Ageing and Human Skill* (1958), which showed that cognitive and sensory-motor performance were improved when older persons had more time to respond. Meanwhile, Harvey Lehman's compilation of creative thinkers in *Age and Achievement* (1953) showed that the intelligence of healthy, active people could improve at least into the seventh decade, longer than previously thought.

Psychologists determined that aged people's aptitude should not be measured by the same instruments used to assess that of young people. IQ tests and Scholastic Aptitude Tests were time specific; older people on average got lower scores because they responded to questions more slowly. Multiple-choice tests did not capture life's choices for them. With fewer years of schooling on average than youth, older people were reluctant to compete in institutional settings that put a premium on mastering skills by rote.

Recent studies of wisdom in late life shed additional light on how people process information and sensations with advancing years. Paul Baltes and his group in Berlin, for instance, differentiate between cognitive mechanics and cognitive pragmatics. This corresponds to the distinction they draw between "fluid" and "crystallized" intelligence. The "software of the mind," hypothesizes the Baltes group, enables some elderly individuals to develop an expert knowledge system, a set of procedures for going about the business of living. In her theory about the nature and engagement of "wise persons," on the other hand, Monika Ardelt acknowledges the importance of cognition but also includes feelings and actions. The thoughts, emotions, and deeds of wise elders, contends Ardelt, ripen purposively and synchronically.

The Baltes group and Ardelt highlight different facets of "wisdom" as a complex, elusive concept. The former assert that wisdom is practical, applicable to everyday situations. The Baltes group stress wisdom's domain specificity: older people can learn skills that make them experts in identifying critical issues and deploying appropriate tools for accomplishing a particular task. Ardelt's paradigm is broader, more spiritually grounded than pragmatic. It is universal in scope, unbounded by time. That these models represent the state of the art tells us something fresh about adult learning (Achenbaum, 2004).

To reach senior citizens, a new orientation using different learning approaches was required. Martin Knowles, a major architect of "modern" theories of adult learning, distinguished between pedagogy and andragogy: "Adults need to know why they need to learn something; adults maintain the contact of responsibility for their own decisions, their own lives; adults enter the educational activity with greater volume and more varied experiences than do children; adults have a readiness to learn those things that they need to know in order to cope effectively with real-life situations; adults are life-centered in their orientation to learning; and adults are more responsive to internal motivators than external motivators" (Knowles et al., 1998: 72; see also Yorks and Kasl, 2002; Rogers, 1995).

Andragogy designed to empower elders through experiential learning necessitates changes in traditional classroom practices. Lesson plans give way to open-ended, expansive discursiveness. Lecturing disadvantages older learners with poor hearing. Instructors must encourage elderly students to integrate new knowledge into their existing cognitive base; rote memorization is not effective. Researchers take account of gender differences: older men generally have immediate, instrumental learning objectives, whereas women consider various options as they map out their course of study. Thus, teachers serve more effectively as facilitators than as fonts of wisdom. They encourage students to design their own curricula, ones that fit their needs (Schleppegrell, 1987: 2; Usher et al., 1997: 23, 43; Naylor, 1999: 3; Hiemstra, 1993: 2–3). Disseminating new directions in adult learning, Jossey-Bass publishes over a hundred monographs on various philosophical and strategic issues in continuing education.

Who constitutes the target population of older learners? A 1995–96 Elderlearning Survey mailed to people between the ages of 55 and 96 who had participated in some study or travel group (mostly under the auspices of Elderhostel) defined some of the parameters. Two thirds of the older learners were women, half of whom were married and a quarter widowed. Roughly 80 percent were between 65 and 80. Although the respondents' income distribution was fairly widely spread, only a quarter reported incomes over $60,000 per year. Older learners strikingly diverged from their age peers in three ways: nearly all were white, at least four-fifths of those between 65 and 89 reported their health to be "excellent" or "good," and committed adult learners had more years of formal schooling than their peers—though the percentages declined with advancing years (Lamdin, 1997: 67–73; for an international comparison, see Ohsako, 1998). The current wave of older learners has advantages their age peers often lack.

According to the National Center for Education Statistics (2002: v, 3), the percent of Americans over the age of 16 who participated in some sort of formal learning program—such as adult basic education, English as a Second Language, and retraining curricula—nearly doubled to 40 percent between 1962 and 1999. More modest increases occurred among those aged 55–64 and among those over age 65. What indeed is most notable is the sharp drop-off in engagement of the two oldest groups compared to all younger cohorts. A trivial percentage of older Americans in 1999 participated in credentialing programs (1.6%, compared to 23.2% for those between the ages of 25 and 34), work-related classes (3.9%, compared to 29.8% for those between 45 and 54), and courses for pleasure—more than a fifth of all Americans between 16 and 54 participated in a non-work-related program compared to 17.3 percent of those between 55 and 64 and 14 percent of those over 65 (ibid.: 71.3).

Learners' preferences vary by age. Younger people are attracted to adult basic education because they think economic advantages will accrue from investing the time. Although older cohorts might wish to compensate for lower levels of educational attainment, they see fewer benefits from participating. Labor-force status and income help to explain elderly people's lack of interest in work-related courses: taking courses does not dramatically alter their prospects for employability. Why are older Americans' participation rates so low in non-work-related courses? Apparently, the offerings do not meet potential interests or needs (ibid.: 29, 45, 50).

Institutional factors also play a role. Although roughly a quarter of those who responded to the Elderlearning Survey reported no barriers to their education, "time" is a big impediment for many. Many elders are busy enjoying retirement, filling their days with volunteering, traveling, and socializing with family and friends. Some who would be interested in taking classes in their community complain that they are not informed about course offerings, sites, and schedules. Others lack the credentials needed to register. Community colleges and most other institutions of higher learning do not reach out to the nation's oldest citizens. The former are primarily concerned with vocational training; the formal degree programs offered by the latter are less appealing to older than younger markets (Lamdin, 1997: 81–82, 92–93; Kett, 1994: 428). Nor are educational centers alone in overlooking older Americans: the 1992 National Adult Literacy Survey paid little attention to men and women over 65, despite the fact that a quarter of that age group scored at the lowest level of proficiency (OVAE, 2004).

It would seem that, despite a fresh understanding of how aged people learn, institutionally we remain stuck where John Dewey drew a blank: opportunities for late-life learners are paltry compared to the programs designed for adults in their prime. Perhaps that inference is myopic. Looking primarily at programs for older adults that fit within traditional modules of higher education may cause us to miss the genuine opportunities for older learners in other contexts. Best practices sometimes develop outside "formal" adult education initiatives. Occasionally they are variations on older ideas formulated in universities. "A curricular focus [that satisfies older learners] within adult learning needs to take account of a lifelong learning process which takes place on multiple sites, acknowledges different identities, celebrates cultural diversity and makes room for all voices," claim Robin Usher and colleagues in *Adult Education and the Postmodern Challenge* (1997: 49).

The United States has not yet replicated Europe's free-standing universities of the Third Age designed for learners at advanced ages, but analogs exist. Nearly half of the students enrolled in St. Mary's School of Economics and Business Administration in California are older students pursuing business skills on a part-time basis (Bole, 1997). Eckert College in Florida erected retirement housing on campus to encourage senior citizens to take courses and to interact with younger students. Rather than build new sites, some institutions are adapting an experiment undertaken in Flint, Michigan, in the 1930s: senior citizens share space with elementary school children, thereby creating a multipurpose educational facility (Sullivan, 2002). The University of North Carolina–Charlotte incorporates service-learning projects for senior citizens taking traditional curricula (Peacock et al., 2001). Bowdoin College in Brunswick, Maine, permits townspeople to participate in campus events for $25 a year. Most colleges and universities sponsor seminars and guided tours for their alumni and friends (Lamdin, 1997: 97). Wesleyan University in Connecticut is building a center to enable emeriti faculty to continue scholarly activities on campus (Wasch, 2004).

Arguably the most imaginative andragogical arrangement to date has been the partnership formed in 1988 between the University of North Carolina at Asheville and the learner-driven North Carolina Center for Creative Retirement. Participants take classes that they design, conduct intergenerational programs to develop leadership skills, and analyze problems in the community and at the state level. Center members compiled a reference work on and for seniors in the United States, *Older Americans Almanac* (1994), which remains as comprehensive and accurate as any scholarly equivalent—and surely more readable (Manheimer, 1994: 738–39).

A fruitful venue for late-life learners likely will be distance education, the latter-day equivalent of the Chautauqua Institution's home-study program. An icon of postmodernity, it reorganizes social relations across large spatial and broad temporal distances and emphasizes "the reflexive appropriation of knowledge," at once unstable and energizing (Giddens, 1990: 53). Tutorial learning with computers satisfies the profile of mature learners eager to maximize available resources for their own purposes. As the success of Britain's Open University (founded in 1971) suggests, a computer-based team approach gives 70-year-olds a "second chance" (Tunstall, 1974: 102) through negotiable but structured interactions. Technologies afford older persons the opportunity to integrate several lines of inquiry, individually or in contact with other learners in educational "chat rooms." Distance education is affordable (administrative overhead is nominal, faculty costs less than on a traditional campus), accessible any time and place, and adaptable enough to link a variety of institutional capacities to meet instructional needs (Keegan, 1993: 28, 166; Bork, 2001; Place et al., 2003: 535).

Several institutions of higher learning, ranging from the University of Illinois to Southern New Hampshire University, have invested heavily in distance education. The University of Wisconsin's Whitewater campus offers an online M.B.A. program (geteducated, 2004). The University of Phoenix is the largest purveyor of online learning. Since its inception in 1976, it has established 128 campuses with Internet delivery worldwide. Roughly 200,000 working professionals have earned degrees by completing a self-paced course that fits their schedules (University of Phoenix, 2002). eCollege.com represents a variation on the Phoenix model; 120 colleges and universities have formed a partnership to offer courses and degrees over the Internet (SeniorCitizens.com, 2004). Because adults over 65 were expected to account for 20 percent of all new online users between 1999 and 2004, and 37 percent of all older persons claimed that continuing education was part of their retirement plans, mature learners may finally attract the attention that their numbers and interest deserve (CenterPoint, 2001).

In their efforts to serve adult learners, leaders of higher education have acknowledged for some time that they operate under budgetary constraints and resistance from other constituencies. Attempts to reach out and to form partnerships in the community have not always been successful. For instance, H. R. Moody, a former president of Elderhostel, the world's largest educational travel organization for men and women over 55, points out that "lack of overheads received, low levels of earnings retained and absence of public funding attached to what is, in effect, a voluntary movement means that educational institutions can only be interested in Elderhostel programmes as a consumer product" (quoted in Walker, 1996: 20–21; see also Elderhostel, 2004). Earlier, a president of the University of Chicago proposed a different way of doing business: "The task of adult education in America today is too broad to be completed by the relatively limited resources of the colleges and universities . . . a university cannot discharge itself of its obligation to adult education merely by the multiplication of its course offerings or the quantitative extension of its program [but] if the job is to be done on a national scale, the universities and colleges must take the lead in the planning of the program" (quoted in Burns and Houle, 1948: 3). Distance learning requires institutional partners: educators plan curricula and andragogies that otherwise autonomous entities implement.

Independent distance-education programs for older people thrive as elderly people become more comfortable with computer-based technologies. A prime example is SeniorNet, launched by the Markle Foundation in 1986. This nonprofit organization provides men and women over 50 with access and training in computer technologies so that they can write autobiographies, construct genealogies, do desktop publishing, and engage in educational projects as well as conduct practical tasks such as managing their personal finances on the Internet. SeniorNet also offers Web courses in Latin, narrative poetry, and reading guides to the sciences. Relying on senior volunteers to coach students in 240 learning sites in community centers, libraries, and clinics in the United States and around the world, SeniorNet has supported millions of older people in collaborative lifelong learning and cross-generational educational experiences (SeniorNet, 2004a, 2004b; geteducated.com, 2004).

Corporate America relies on e-learning as an integral part of their training programs for older workers and retirees. Men and women between 50 and 84, the fastest-growing user group, require on average twice as long to become comfortable with computer-based programs as those between the ages of 20 and 39, but they achieve comparable performance levels. Corporations, guided by university-based researchers in adult learning, often develop community partnerships to provide training information, family counseling, and longer-term assistance because it facilitates the learning process of older workers proceeding at their own pace. Employers claim that distance education is cost-efficient, par-

ticularly as economic downturns mandate cutbacks in corporate training budgets (learnframe, 2001; memletics, 2004; EricDigests, 1991: 3;
EricDigests, 1995: 3; see also, chapter 2 above). Public agencies contribute: Precinct 3 of the Houston-based Area Agency on Aging, for instance, has dedicated considerable space in its new facilities and hired
instructors to offer its elderly constituents basic e-mail classes and advanced training in designing spreadsheets. Computer technologies enable
trainers to overcome language and geographic barriers in reaching culturally diverse participants in the international marketplace.

The federal government encourages civil servants and their families
to use distance education resources. Foreign Service officers based in the
Washington, D.C., area can pursue traditional degrees, noncredit programs, and correspondence courses using computers in libraries and
colleges as well as through professional associations and independent
organizations. Those overseas have access to virtually the same resources
through the Internet. The U.S. Department of Agriculture offers a host
of computer-based graduate-level courses. Their programs are linked to
distance education centers, including the University of Missouri–Columbia, e-learners, and the Indiana Higher Education Telecommunication
System Distance Education Resources (U.S. Department of State, 2004).

Libraries, acquiring new computer technologies, have begun to reach
out to older learners. According to Diantha Schull, president of Libraries
for the Future, "as librarians become aware of the growing numbers of
elders who do not fit the stereotypical associations of aging with illness
and decline, they are recognizing the need to rethink the purposes, scope,
and content of services for people age 50 and over" (Schull, 2004). A
1998 survey of 625 public libraries in Pennsylvania, for instance, revealed that a quarter of the users were between the ages of 35 and 44.
Retirees constituted roughly another quarter of those served. Women
represented more than 70 percent of the patrons. While some older persons yearned for card catalogs, they have proven as receptive as younger
patrons to learning new techniques. Librarians and tutors instruct older
people in how to email their grandchildren and friends, monitor their
investments, visit Web sites dealing with their hobbies, and check electronic bulletin boards to learn about cultural events and volunteer opportunities. Public libraries have introduced more than a quarter of its
patrons to new technologies; a tenth of those sampled said that they sub-
sequently bought computers and subscribed to Internet accounts for use

in their homes (McClure and Bertot, 1998: 57, 61; Ore Module, 2004; Simon, 2004: 2).

Besides assisting with computer-based instruction, public libraries sponsor volunteer activities. With support from state grants, libraries are able to recruit older adults as tutors, mentors, and program developers. A few examples suggest the range of activities. The Santa Monica [Calif.] Public Library and the Waterford [Mich.] Public Library select and deliver books of interest to the homebound and those in nursing homes. The Beauregard Parish [La.] Public Library sends an outreach team with a "traveling museum" to prompt interactions in senior centers and adult day care sites. A 25-member consortium of libraries in San Francisco formed "The Bay Area Literacy Initiative" to enable older adults to assist their peers in improving their reading and writing skills. That some older Americans easily bridge self-learning projects with commitments as volunteers suggests a fruitful avenue to adult learning: in making time to serve others, older Americans learn skills useful to their own needs and development.

Volunteering as a Way of Applying Lifelong Learning

Although indifference and structural lags have limited the access of older Americans to continuing education, senior citizens play a critical role as volunteers in the United States. According to the Bureau of Labor Statistics (2004: Tables 1 and 4), slightly more than a quarter of all citizens over 16 do unpaid work through one or two organizations. Whites, women, and those with at least some college education are most likely to volunteer. The percentage of those between the ages of 55 and 64 engaged in volunteer activities is slightly above the national average (29.2%), those over 65 slightly below (23.7%). It is important to note that the very old contribute the most. The median annual hours (88) contributed by the oldest cohort far exceeded the 52 hours given by all other age groups. Older persons cite an enhanced sense of purpose, personal growth, and a feeling of productiveness as reasons for volunteering (Bradley, 1999–2000).

Mature adults on average volunteer to religious institutions and civic groups. Significantly, the percentages of volunteers over 55 who contribute to social service and community-based projects exceeds the general population. According to the 2000 NCOA survey of Myths and

Realities of Aging, nearly 40 percent of older respondents involved in community service felt that their efforts enabled them to reclaim their place in society (Cutler, Whitelaw, and Beattie, 2002; Keyser, 2003; Dahlberg, 2004). There is room for even greater engagement by older people to serve as volunteers in civic agencies that traditionally relied on the altruism of younger persons.

The untapped potential to facilitate older Americans in applying their experiential learning and expertise has not been lost on social commentators. Horace Deets, former executive director of AARP, believes that "as a public issue, we must look at the aging of society and figure out how to incorporate the longevity bonus into our planning and policies. If we don't find ways to allow people to continue making contributions to society as they get older, an older, dependent population will become a self-fulfilling prophecy. This planning requires a systems approach to understand how all the parts fit together. All the elements need to be in alignment along the continuum of life and across the public and private sectors" (Deets, 2001). Senior citizens are integral to "bridging [that] social capital" essential to rebuilding communities and to cultivating networks at the local, national, and global levels. Thanks to extra healthful years, elders have the time that is needed to build relational trust and mutual understanding (Putnam and Feldstein, 2003: 3, 5, 13). Researchers find that very old adults feel personal satisfaction and self-respect as they help others. It is part of their legacy (Bukov et al., 2002; *Generations*, 1996: 66; Mentors Peer Services, 2004).

The history of OASIS, the nation's largest and most comprehensive educational and volunteer service program designed for senior citizens, presents an exemplary case study of how to build a multidimensional resource for active, productive older adults who want to do good by staying active. OASIS was conceived in 1982 by Marylen Mann and Margie Wolcott May with seed money from the U.S. Administration on Aging and classroom space donated by the May department stores. At the end of the two-year demonstration projects conducted in St. Louis, Baltimore, Cleveland, and Los Angeles, OASIS forged partnerships with local sponsors in other cities to develop intergenerational tutoring programs and to launch wellness programs with hospitals and other health providers. In addition to support from the May Company, the National Endowment for the Humanities, and the Emerson and SBC foundations, May piloted initiatives in mentoring, its HealthStages program, humanities projects, and the use of the Internet to connect senior citizens to other opportunities and projects. The Robert Wood Johnson Foundation gave OASIS a million dollars in 2003 for its Active for Life Program. OASIS currently serves 350,000 mature adults in 26 cities "to continue their personal growth and provide meaningful service to the community" (OASIS, 2003).

The federal government has sponsored public-private volunteerism under its own aegis. Senior Corps (2004a, 2004b, 2004c) oversees three important programs:

- *The Retired and Senior Volunteer Program* (RSVP) recruits approximately 480,000 citizens over 55 to serve in 65,000 nonprofit organizations, public agencies, and faith-based institutions. Volunteers monitor neighborhood watch groups, mentor youth at risk, teach English to immigrants, and test drinking water, among other things.
- *Foster Grandparents* provides positions for 30,000 people over 60 with limited incomes to address the needs of young mothers and abused children, including those with physical disabilities, in schools; correctional facilities; Head Start, drug treatment, and day-care centers; and hospitals.
- *The Senior Companion Program* (SCP), a spin-off of Foster Grandparents, appeals to the compassion of 15,500 aged, low-income volunteers to assist the frail elderly and homebound in completing daily tasks and monitoring on a one-on-one basis the health status of the person they are assisting.

Two examples will suffice to illustrate the other federal initiatives that exist. Among the several supported by the U.S. Administration on Aging is the Senior Medicare Patrol launched in 1997, which has trained more than 48,000 retired doctors, nurses, accountants, and attorneys to help Medicaid and Medicare beneficiaries become better consumers by understanding the complexities of the programs, preventing billing errors, and identifying potential fraud. The U.S. Small Business Administration sponsors a 13,000-member association of retired executives and owners (SCORE) to counsel men and women as they start up and manage new ventures (U.S. Administration on Aging, 2004).

The compassion and commitments of older Americans are also being used in the nation's public school system. With more and more mothers in the labor force, older people assume roles as school volunteers. The

National School Volunteer Program begun in 1986 started filling the gap. So did local initiatives, including North Carolina's Agelink, started in 1990, an intergenerational child-care program that linked older Americans with children in after-school programs, and Salt Lake City's Senior Motivators in Learning and Educational Services (SMILES), which helped with field trips, reading, and sports (Lipson, 1994; Sullivan, 2002).

Currently, Experience Corps is the most important organization deploying the time and energy of older Americans in the classroom. Like OASIS, good leadership, foundation and governmental funding, strong community support, and incremental implementation turned a good idea into reality. John Gardner, the 80-year-old former secretary of Health, Education, and Welfare, proposed in a three-page paper the notion that men and women in their third age were in the enjoyable and enviable position of making important contributions to societal well-being. The Commonwealth Foundation invited Marc Freedman, a baby boomer social entrepreneur, to draft a concept paper with the help of his mentor, John Gardner. Freedman's ideas about ways to tap the expertise of elderly people in understaffed classrooms for disadvantaged children were based on his travels and the innovations created by the Foster Grandparents Programs. In his report, Freedman emphasized that the Experience Corps had to be a serious enterprise, requiring serious commitment from volunteers and a critical mass of workers so that they could have an impact not only on the schools but also on the local community (Freedman, 1983; Freedman, 1999: 178–83). Mobilizing people into a workable program was not easy, however.

Institutions must provide the public and private underwriting as well as the technical assistance that are critical to the task. AARP helped to identify enough initial volunteers for Experience Corps to constitute a critical mass. Potential tutors were given the option of full-time work (thanks to a surplus of workers available through VISTA), twenty hours a week of service through Experience Corps, or part-time (two hours, two days a week) or episodic (seasonal) posts. The profile of volunteers in North Philadelphia gives a good indication of what Experience Corps sought: they were largely healthy, vital African-American women considerably over 50, who were mainly former teachers and public employees. They were trained—although some were weeded out—at Temple University's Center for Intergenerational Learning. Results were impressive: after two years the reading scores of three-quarters of those taught by Experience Corps teachers rose by one grade level. Anecdotal evidence suggests other benefits. Students took more pride in themselves and were more hopeful about the future; they learned lessons in civility; they profited from a school environment enriched by older people who cared (Freedman, 1999: 213; Putnam and Feldstein, 2003: 201, 203). With support from the Robert Wood Johnson Foundation and Atlantic Philanthropies, Experience Corps is expanding beyond its five pilot studies and recruiting more volunteers.

Other intergenerational educational programs merit notice. Sally Newman at the University of Pittsburgh mobilized senior citizens to prepare preschool children for formal education. Taking cues from the Foxfire project, researchers at Georgia Institute of Technology use computer technology to enable students to address questions about "living history" to those who served in World War II and in the civil rights movement. Computers also make it possible to transcend the generation gap as fourth-graders develop friendships and learning experiences with nursing-home residents in Ohio (Ellis et al., n.d.; Jobe, 1999). Some projects target special populations in need. Beverly Benner Cassara, a professor of adult education in Washington, D.C., started an educational program in low-income housing to educate African-American women. Fourteen women in the first cohort earned general educational diplomas (Hall of Fame, 2003). Octogenarians in Peoria volunteer their time to tutor students with learning disabilities. Linking Lifetimes uses mentors over 55 in nine states to help to rehabilitate juvenile offenders (Dagostino, 1997; Rogers, 1995; Lipson, 1994). Parent Aide Project (started in 1988 by AARP) conjoins senior citizens with parents to serve as role models in rescuing children at risk. The project also helps school officials train older volunteers to deal with child abuse and neglect (Penn State, 1988).

*Intra*generational projects attract less attention but merit discussion. I will discuss caregiving opportunities for elders helping elders in greater depth in the next chapter, but here the role minorities play in volunteerism is worth note. Ninety-year-old African Americans like Anselmo Marshall are viewed as a "godsend" in the Central Harlem Senior Citizens Center because of their willingness, after training with the Retired Senior Volunteer Program, to assist residents with performing their daily tasks (Haskell, 2004). Elders help in other ways. SHINE (Serving Health

Insurance Needs of Elders) invites men and women over 60 to help other senior citizens with making claims and appeals, comparing policies, and doing the paperwork (Wilson, 1994). Volunteers in Medicine and Samaritan House represent two clinics staffed by volunteer healthcare professionals who demonstrate ways to engage in healthcare reform as they attend to the medical needs of older patients (Freedman 1999, 148–49). Doula (Greek for "grief") teams senior volunteers with terminally ill patients who would otherwise die alone (Kleinfield, 2004a: 1, 20).

Some mature citizens volunteer for groups that espouse wider horizons than neighborhood senior centers or local elementary schools. "The Community Without Walls" did a pilot study of volunteerism among men and women over 55 for thirteen charitable and nonprofit organizations in the Princeton, New Jersey, area. They found that 406 volunteers, of whom two-thirds were retired, contributed 35,147 hours (the dollar equivalent of $1.4 million) in 2002 to giving assistance to animal shelters, the YMCA, and schools; doing clerical work in congressional district offices; and counseling in the Crisis Ministry of Princeton and Trenton. Most groups expected to expand their geographical sphere of activities as they trained more volunteers (Community Without Walls, 2003: 3). Environmental issues attract some older volunteers. Since 1997 more than a thousand members of Pennsylvania's Senior Environmental Corps, with funds from the state's departments of aging and environmental protection and a Virginia-based nonprofit organization, have examined stream banks for erosion and measured the conductivity, alkalinity, and acidity of the commonwealth's waterways (May, 2001). Emulating Jimmy and Rosalynn Carter, older people have also participated in Habitat for Humanity, traveling in vans to build homes for low-income persons in one community after the next (Freedman, 1999: ix, 234; Dahlberg, 2004: 47). Organizations that originally recruited undergraduates and men and women just out of college—such as Big Brother/Big Sister, the YMCA, and the Peace Corps—now increasingly solicit volunteers over 55.

What might entice an even greater percentage of older Americans to volunteer their time? Several proposals could easily be implemented. Like anyone else, senior volunteers need constructive feedback for their efforts. Some want a title, authorization to perform prescribed tasks and participate in the fulfillment of specific strategies, or an appointment to organizational committees—all of which make them feel that they are a

valued part of the organization. More importantly, they want assignments that challenge their minds and fulfill their sense of purpose. Jack
Hexter, who moved to Washington University when he was forced to
retire from Yale, knew this. At 80, anticipating the reduction of army
forces after the Gulf War, he proposed "Troops for Teachers," targeting
African-American and Latino soldiers from the inner city to become certified teachers. Senator John Danforth championed the program, which
placed more than 3,000 retired veterans in the forty-eight contiguous
states but mainly in Texas, Florida, California, and Virginia (Freedman,
1999: 164; *Prevention,* 1999; *Journal of Extension,* 1992; Kieffer, 1986).
Saluting the time and effort of elderly volunteers is an important moti-
vator. Hence, the MetLife Foundation honors annually twenty-five volunteers over 55 for their team spirit, mentoring, and community leadership (Association for Volunteer Administration, 2004).

Volunteers obviously do not expect to be paid for their contributions,
but most would like some assistance in covering their expenses. Service
credits for helping others in hospitals, health maintenance organizations,
religious communities, and housing complexes might be cashed in when
the volunteers need them (Tseng and Mueller, 2001). Funds should be
allocated to agencies too small to be able to afford the cost of liability
insurance (Fischer and Schaffer, 2004). And just as adult learners might
be permitted to draw on their Social Security contributions to pay for
training at mid-career, so too it would not be unreasonable to give older
people who care for children and elders some credit for their activities
as a way to decrease their income tax liability.

To provide more incentives for volunteering, we need more funds and
a better sense of what makes men and women satisfied and satisfying as
volunteers. It seems churlish to ask private philanthropies to contribute
more, given what they have done so far, but it is clear that recruiting
senior citizens to engage in productive activities, including volunteering,
becomes a high priority when child welfare is at stake. U.S. grantmak-
ing institutions gave $4.46 billion to benefit children and youth in 2001,
double the amount granted in 1996. The creation of the Bill & Melinda
Gates Foundation, which immediately became the prime benefactor in
2000, coupled with a bull market, made such largesse possible (Lawrence, 2002).

In contrast, foundations that support productive aging tend to be
smaller and quite specific in earmarking funds. The Atlantic Philan-

thropies, for instance, is spending down its $3.9 billion endowment as it focuses on four issues: aging, disadvantaged children and youth, the health problems of developing countries, and reconciliation and human rights. This is consistent with Atlantic's mission—"to bring lasting changes that will improve the lives of disadvantaged and vulnerable people"—but it limits grantmaking in aging to Bermuda, Northern Ireland, the Republic of Ireland, and the United States (Atlantic Philanthropies, 2003). The Gerontological Society of America (2003), among other groups, updates Web sites that fund research and services on aging. Foundation heads and consultants meet regularly under the aegis of Grantmakers in Aging to brainstorm and bolster institutional commitments (Grantmakers in Aging, 2004).

Besides more funding, we need a better sense of what personal attributes make some older volunteers readily and effectively assume leadership roles as mentors. Some data are available from organizations that help elderly people refine the talents that they possess. Linking learning and volunteering in diverse institutional settings may increase the pool of potential volunteers willing and able to contribute to improving the circumstances of children and youth.

Mentoring as a Service to Humanity

Just as not all men and women grow wiser with advancing years, not all adult learners and volunteers have the aptitude or experiences to be mentors. It is a legacy of mentors, as Greek mythology relates in the relationship between Mentor and Telemachus (Hornblower and Spawforth, 1996: 961), to listen carefully to a younger person's goals and then to help the mentee in appropriate ways to journey toward success and to deal with the contingencies of life, so that in due course he or she may mentor another person. Mentoring takes on diverse forms—short term/long term, focused/serendipitous, team/individual—to meet people's different needs (Search Institute, 1995; Conway, 1998). Baby boomers, especially members of ethnic and racial minorities and women, benefit from the counsel and experience of an elder who knows the ethos and standard operating procedures of an institutional setting (*Aging Today*, 1998; Saito and Roehlkepartain, 1992; Conway, 1998; Center for Third Age Leadership, 2004).

Corporations tap their retired executives to help promising middle-managers rise through the ranks. For example, in 1987 Egemin started to recruit laid-off older workers to share their experiences and knowledge with younger people; there is now one person over 48 for every ten workers under that age on the payroll (Egemin Worldwide, 2004). A 1999 survey of 636 mentor-mentee relationships in national and multinational companies revealed that 42 percent of the pairings were designed to promote career development, 30 percent were targeted for technology transfer, and 12 percent to deal with issues of cultural diversity (American Society of Aging, 1999; Murray, 2001: 31).

Mentors have been important in upgrading science education in public schools. Sometimes they work directly with students and sometimes with teachers, principals, and superintendents. Unlike tutors, mentors serving in this capacity are typically backed by a company (such as Hewlett Packard or the Merck Institute for Science Education) or a professional organization (such as the American Chemical Society or the Society of Automotive Engineers) or a university (such as Northeastern or the California Institute of Technology) that wants to improve young people's literacy and to stir the imaginations of the older persons (National Academies of Science, 2004; Parsons, 1999).

Once again, foundations have played a crucial part in creating a niche for older adults. Convinced that many youth had lost their "natural proximity to caring, mature adults," the Commonwealth Fund's Margaret Mahoney began to underwrite mentoring programs in the 1980s. One of the first projects, which involved matching one hundred mature black women with disadvantaged youth, became the basis for Career Beginnings (Freedman, 1993: 3). More recently, Atlantic Philanthropies gave the National Council on the Aging $3.4 million to identify the structural barriers that impede civic engagement in late life. Additional support came from the MetLife Foundation to empower senior citizens to work in this area (Reilly, 2003: 10).

Mentors are needed in virtually all domains: coaching, working in communities with youth, developing entrepreneurial skills, marketing, designing alternative educational programs, and assisting new professionals (Freedman, 1993: 92). Mentors Peer Services, a Canadian concern, maintains a Web site of companies, agencies, churches, schools, and other organizations that use mentors (2004). Most of the listings are small organizations in North America or Britain. But thanks to the Internet, older adults can find out what is available as easily and quickly as they can retrieve information about adult learning and volunteering. Advances in computer technology hold forth the possibility of older people taking a structural lead in broadening opportunities to engage instead of being marginalized by structural lags.

There is one final area of growth in which only a few older individuals discover that they have the talent and experience to ripen. Creativity has elements of learning, volunteering, and mentoring, but it is a gift *sui generis*. Creativity requires the discerning eye, the deft touch, the expert's mastery to know if, where, and when a product (artistic, literary, or scientific) should be brought to fruition. Creativity requires perseverance and curiosity, a willingness to take risks that make sense because the creative person has learned well from prior successes and failures. Mentors, peers, and youth can help older persons to be creative by encouraging them to take risks and by allaying their fears of failure (Carlsen, 1991; Kerka, 1999). Age, once considered to be antithetical to creativity, now seems to be but one factor that affects the production of novel ways of thinking and seeing. Experience utilized in late life matters more than has been previously recognized.

In the end, the wellspring of creativity lies within an individual's dogged determination and ability to make sense out of chaos, to glean truth from a serendipitous occurrence. Creativity is domain specific: mathematicians and bench scientists tend to peak earlier than historians and philosophers. Some creative people work in the same medium all their lives, others switch once or twice, and still others develop a new interest after ending a successful career. There is no single pathway to important discoveries, but with the longevity revolution underway, we may predict that more and more innovations will be made in all realms of science and culture by creative people over 60 (Simonton, 1988; Csikszentmihalyi, 1995; Galenson, 2003).

On the basis of her study of 150 well-known people between the ages of 65 and 101, all of whom engaged in some sort of creative activity in late life, Lydia Bronte concluded:

> The study participants confirmed the importance of a continuing and renewed sense of responsibility in the lives of older people. Many of them relished the fact that their personal responsibilities had diminished, whereas their more global responsibilities were expanding. They finally had the time and the financial security to direct their ener-

gies in making broader contributions; in addition, they now had the experience and wisdom that make their contributions most valuable. Moreover, although most of them did not say so explicitly, it was suggested that the older decades had brought them a sense of increasing altruism. They were genuinely concerned about the needs of their communities. They sought out certain activities, not to satisfy their egos or to prove that they could still "cut the mustard," but because they wanted to see the quality of human life improve. (Bronte, 1993: 298–99)

Bronte's study takes us full circle. John Dewey lived in an era in which most experts thought that the decrements of age were inevitable. Social planners in the 1930s discounted what older people could contribute. Bronte, based on an admittedly unique survey of creatively impressive senior citizens, nonetheless documents that extra years make vital careers possible, ones that enrich the lives of elderly persons and those whose lives they touch. Few of us will attain the stature or make the accomplishments of a Hume Cronyn, "Mother" Clara Hale, Elizabeth Janeway, or Dr. Jonas Salk. But contributions made by ordinary men and women as learners, volunteers, and mentors are sufficient to give hope that, as the baby boomer generation ages, it too will be at least as inquisitive, altruistic, and vital as the cohort that preceded it.

4 { Reforming the U.S. Health System to Care for an Aging Population

William Osler (1849–1919) was arguably the Anglo-American scientific community's preeminent physician at the beginning of the twentieth century. After teaching at McGill University and the University of Pennsylvania, he was recruited in 1888 to head the Johns Hopkins Hospital as well as to serve as a professor of medicine in the university's planned school of medicine. In this dual role, Osler revolutionized medical curricula in North America, adapting the best German research and British clinical practices to patient care. His textbook, *The Principles and Practice of Medicine* (1892), became the *classicus locus* for the next forty years (Johns Hopkins Health System, 1999).

In 1905, Dr. Osler accepted the Regius Professorship of Medicine at Oxford, academic medicine's most prestigious position at the time. In his valedictory address to his colleagues, students, and friends at Johns Hopkins, Osler offered "two fixed ideas well known to my friends": "The first is the comparative uselessness of men above forty years of age. . . . In the science and art of medicine young or comparatively young men have made every advance of the first rank. . . . The young men should be encouraged and afforded every possible chance to show what is in them. . . . My second fixed idea is the uselessness of men above sixty years of age, and the incalculable benefit it would be in commercial, political and in professional life if, as a matter of course, men stopped work at this age" (quoted in Graebner, 1980: 4–5).

At 56, Dr. Osler knew all too well "from studying sclerotic arteries and deteriorating organs in the dead house" the course of pathological lesions that weakened men at 40 and rendered workers twenty years older virtually obsolescent. Whereas in the first edition of *The Principles and Practices of Medicine,* he had called pneumonia "the special enemy of old age," by the third edition (1898), Osler judged it "the friend of the aged." Pneumonia, opined Dr. Osler, alleviated at last the "cold gradations of decay" (Bliss, 1999: 290, 327, 501).

Healthcare professionals' disesteem for old people did not begin with Dr. Osler's generation. Negativity toward old people dates back to ancient times. In the fourteenth of his *Precepts,* Hippocrates declared that "the prime of life has everything lovely, the decline has the opposite" (trans. Jones, 1948: 1:331). There were exceptions to unflattering portraits of senescence over time. The factors contributing to the prolongation of human life fascinated medical practitioners and investigators from one century to the next (Gruman, 2003). For instance, Benjamin Rush enjoyed caring for the Founding Fathers as they entered their ninth decade, including those who lost their mental faculties and physical strength (Achenbaum, 1978a: 14; Cole, 1992: 103). Subsequent advances in medical knowledge, technology, and surgical procedures reinforced prejudices, however. Rejecting Rush's assumption that old age was basically the result of "natural decay," leading medical scientists in the second half of the nineteenth century utilized new techniques and instrumentation to probe the pathological aspects models of aging. Some went a step further and called old age a disease *sui generis.* To their dismay, no intervention—dietary, surgical, or testicular—retarded and eradicated old people's lesions or curious behavior.

On the eve of World War I, when I. L. Nascher launched geriatrics as a medical subspecialty in the United States by issuing a textbook by that name, he had trouble convincing colleagues that the processes and diseases of late life deserved investigation. (Finding a publisher for *Geriatrics* was also difficult.) As a physician, Nascher noted, one has "a natural reluctance to exert oneself for those who are economically worthless and must remain so, or to strive against the inevitable, though there be the possibility of momentary success, or to devote time and effort in so unfruitful a field when both can be used to greater material advantage in other fields of medicine" (Nascher, 1914: vii–viii). The founder of U.S. geriatrics admitted in 1926 that he was the nation's only full-time practitioner (Achenbaum, 1995b: 47).

Thereafter, interest in geriatrics and gerontology grew, albeit slowly,

United States. The Josiah Macy Jr. Foundation sponsored a land-
conference whose proceedings, edited by Edmund V. Cowdry, appeared in three editions under the title *Problems of Ageing* (1939, 1941;
Lansing, 1952). The Macy Foundation also formed a partnership in
1940 with the U.S. Public Health Service to create a Unit on Gerontology within the National Institutes of Health. The American Geriatrics
Society was chartered in 1942, and the Gerontological Society of America three years later (Achenbaum, 1995b). "The more we know about
the biologic mechanisms of the ageing processes," declared Dr. Edward
Stieglitz, one of the prime movers of research on aging after World War
II, "the more effectively can clinical medicine treat the ageing and the
aged" (Stieglitz, 1943: 906; for British parallels, see Sheldon, 1948).

Despite such efforts to ameliorate the well-being of the elderly population, Dr. Robert Butler, the first director of the National Institute on
Aging, painted a grim picture of elder care in his 1975 Pulitzer Prize–
winning critique, *Why Survive? Being Old in America:* "The bad news
is that the majority of older people can't afford proper medical care; doctors and health personnel are not trained to deal with their unique problems; their medical conditions are not considered interesting to teaching
institutions; and they are stereotyped as bothersome, cantankerous and
complaining patients. Direct prejudices exist" (Butler, 1975: 174). Butler was particularly concerned that healthcare professionals embraced
mainstream culture's animus against age. In 1968 he coined the term
ageism to define "a process of systematic stereotyping of and discrimination against people because they are old, just as racism and sexism
accomplish this with skin color and gender" (quoted in Bernstein, 1968).
Butler was appalled that medical students and their professors described
elderly patients as having "serum porcelain levels"—that is, they were
crocks. Among other terms used were *gomer* (for "get out of my emergency room") and *gork* (for "God only really knows [what's wrong]")
(Butler, 1975: 180; T. Nelson, 2002: 350). Ageism, according to Butler,
was not only an individually held prejudice but was also deeply embed-
ded into the U.S. medical system. Ageism fostered attitudinal and institutional roadblocks to delivering accessible, adequate health care to
older Americans.

The Present State of Ageism in the Healthcare Professions

Since 1975 there have been increases in life expectancy and overall improvements in the healthfulness of the current cohort of senior citizens.
Advances in preventive medicine, public health, and clinical research
bode well for baby boomers and succeeding generations. These salutary
developments might have caused a decline in ageism, just as cultural
currents and public policies have dampened tolerance for racism and
sexism. Alternatively, stereotypes ascribed to adults over 65 (National
Council on the Aging, 1974) might have been pushed back to describe
the health of the old-old. Surprisingly, neither trend has happened.

Nearly three decades after he wrote *Why Survive?* Butler saw "little
change" in the virulence of ageism in the U.S. healthcare system (Pope,
2003). Nor was he alone in this distressing assessment. Medical journals
have published countless reports and editorials documenting that physicians still make erroneous diagnoses and forgo reasonable treatments of
patients 65 and older. Commentators attribute the lackluster performance to the negative or nihilistic attitudes doctors harbor, especially
when compared to their care of young people. Trainees express ageist
sentiments from the time they begin to work on the cadaver of an older
person. More than 80 percent of a group of Johns Hopkins medical students claimed that they would admit to intensive care a 10-year-old girl
with pneumonia and treat her aggressively, whereas only a slight majority of those surveyed reported that they would do the same for an
85-year-old woman (ibid.: 5).

Some researchers hypothesize that physicians do not like older people because, consciously or not, they project onto physiological aging
their own fears of growing older and dying. Ageism among healthcare
practitioners may have psychological aspects, but it also reflects workplace conditions and professional standards. With other patients waiting and the bills of elderly patients not fully reimbursed by Medicare,
some doctors reckon that old people use up too many of their resources.
Health professionals criticize older persons as time consuming and habit-
ual complainers (CBSNews.com, 2004). Unlike younger patients, very
old patients by and large present multiple clinical problems.

The presence of several diseases and chronic conditions can make it
difficult to reach a proper diagnosis and to chart an appropriate course
of treatment for elderly adults. Physical diseases are occasionally mis-

perceived as mental disorders. Physiological changes that may not be pathological in themselves can contribute to declines in physical capacity that can affect the course of disease elsewhere in an aging body. Physicians who do not keep up with recent advances reported in the geriatric literature persist in believing that virtually every decrement associated with senescence is irreversible. In addition to these factors, researchers report that hospital protocols and insurance regulations often impede physicians' ability and willingness to obtain complete personal and medical histories from elderly patients (Safford and Krell, 1992: 52; B. Robinson, 1994; Birren, 1996, 1:77; Carstensen et al., 1996: 168; Armerding, 2002). "Many pitfalls thus stand in the way of correct diagnosis and treatment. Perhaps the greatest of all is stereotyping the elderly patient as the victim of 'aging'" (Reichel, 1978: 17).

Primary care physicians are not the only clinicians who express ageist prejudices. Let us consider the ways that ageist attitudes play themselves out in several dissimilar specialties. Ageism and age-related misconceptions color surgeons' assessments of the risks of performing surgery on patients advancing in years. For instance, two-fifths of the people affected by colorectal cancer are over 75. Typically, because of one or more other existing conditions, nonelective surgical procedures have higher rates of morbidity and mortality than elective surgeries. Yet according to the Apache III system, which looks at the risk factors predicting outcomes among (especially old) intensive-care patients, roughly half the variability in morbidity and mortality is due to the *intensity* of a particular acute illness. Only 3 percent can be attributed to chronological age. Problems with anesthesia pose a far greater risk than advanced age in performing surgery on an octogenarian in otherwise relatively good health (Tallis and Fillit, 2003: 320–21).

Dentists, to take a second example, recognize that oral hygiene is typically given a low priority by health practitioners and older people alike. But maintaining good oral health is essential to promoting healthful aging. Roughly a quarter of men and women between the ages of 65 and 74 have severe periodontal diseases. Older Americans are seven times more likely to be diagnosed with oral cancer than younger people. Epidemiologists have associated the presence of oral infections with diabetes, heart disease, and respiratory problems. Yet few nursing homes and long-term care facilities are equipped to deliver oral health services for their residents, precisely the subgroup of the old-old population most at risk. And because few public or private insurance plans provide dental coverage, elderly Americans, especially those with low incomes, are disinclined to visit their dentists: only 45 percent of those over 75 visited a dentist during the past year, compared to 61 percent of the entire population (Carmona, 2003).

Even osteopaths, whose patients include large numbers of elderly people, acknowledge that their students lack basic competencies for caring for older patients. At the head of their 1998 osteopathic curriculum were recommended proficiencies in attitudes. First came "awareness of the various myths and stereotypes related to older people," followed by "recognition that agism, like racism, affects all levels and aspects of society including health professions and can adversely affect optimal care of elderly patients" (American Geriatrics Society, 1998). Osteopathic medical educators went on to urge students to assess their own attitudes toward aging, to exercise compassion and understanding in dealing with the frail elderly, and to realize that America's aged population, for all its diversity, is composed of individuals who should be "cared for in a unique fashion."

And what about physicians who want to specialize in geriatrics? The relative lack of prestige and financial rewards for geriatricians induces doctors to pursue other specialties and practices. There are presently only 9,000 geriatricians in the United States compared to 42,000 pediatricians. Given the fact that physicians are seeing greater numbers of older people in their practices, it would behoove them to learn about caring for old people in medical school. However, they have few opportunities. A mere 10 percent of the nation's medical schools require course work or rotations in geriatric medicine. Only 5 of the 145 accredited schools have departments of geriatric medicine. Fewer than 3 percent of medical school graduates take electives in geriatrics (Breaux, 2003a).

Physicians' aversion to caring for elderly patients can be gauged in other ways. Allowing for variations in the routines of specialties such as oncology and internal medicine, the average encounter time between patients and their doctors in offices and in hospitals rises slightly among the 55–64 age cohort, then drops significantly after the age of 65. It drops further among patients over 75. Health maintenance organizations and medical centers press their staffs to spend less time with patients, which increases the temptation to engage in stereotyping (Kane et al., 1981: 26–29; Nelson, 2002: 50). Clinicians tend to dominate conversations when dealing with older adults. Studies indicate that they are less respectful, less patient, and less engaged than they are when interacting with younger patients (Carstensen et al., 1996: 168; Quill, 1989a). Cuts in Medicare reimbursements and higher costs of practice, according to the American Medical Association, have resulted in physicians' limiting access to elders, discontinuing certain services, and referring complex cases to specialists or shunting them to teaching hospitals (Alliance for Aging Research, 2003: 4; E. Radin, personal communication, 2004).

Elderly persons also get short shrift in screening for diseases and other health maladies. According to a 2003 Centers for Disease Control and Prevention report, nine out of ten adults over 65 go without appropriate screening. Heart disease is the number one cause of death among elderly people, yet nearly half who had high blood pressure readings did not realize they were hypertensive. Experts disagree about the value of screening for certain diseases, however. The American College of Physicians and the American Society of Internal Medicine recommend against regular mammographies among women over 75. The U.S. Preventive Services Task Force cited insufficient evidence for or against the procedure, claiming that the decision to screen older women should be made on other grounds (Rich and Sox, 2000). Clinical trials for older persons may require the development of different instruments and measures in testing the efficacy of antipsychotic medications on patients with Alzheimer's disease (Lebowitz, 2004). As we shall see below, the debate raises a fundamental issue: Should older people be routinely omitted from clinical trials, despite their being the largest consumers of approved drugs?

Elderly patients, surveys reveal, typically internalize the ageist biases they perceive in their physicians. Some avoid making appointments when they become ill; they forgo annual check-ups. Others neglect to mention aches and pains that might be symptomatic of serious disease (National Center for Health Statistics, 2003: 235). Still others confirm their doctors' expectations: they complain endlessly about minor ailments; they seek as many second and third opinions as their insurance coverage and pocketbooks permit. Despite the adoption in 1957 of "informed consent" to lessen the potential for malpractice suits, many patients report feeling ignored or poorly briefed as they make critical healthcare choices. "Informed consent" has rarely been used as a plaintiff's sole ground for recovery, which some medical ethicists claim indicates that the public either does not know about the principle or views it as weak protection. Finally, age differences between physician and patient have been shown to be a barrier to effective communication, which perforce impairs medical treatment. Studies indicate that a physician's silence surrounding death is often construed by the dying as abandonment (Quill, 1989a; J. Katz, 2002).

Elderly persons often are stigmatized by prejudicial words and deeds expressed by other members of their healthcare team. Nurses tend to rate their aged patients as more dysfunctional than indicated by objective measures. Here and abroad, studies indicate that student nurses view older people predominantly as frail and as declining in health. Nurses say that they find older patients uninteresting. It takes more time to accomplish routine tasks for them (Palmore, 1999: 147). No wonder children, relatives, and friends typically render more accurate assessments of older patients than those who work in hospitals and nursing homes (M. B. Miller, 1979: 17; Carstensen et al., 1996: 157; Moyle, 2002). Many nurses simply have not been trained and are not motivated to grapple with aged people's chronic ailments. Pediatrics remains a mainstay of nursing school programs; few institutions offer geriatric concentrations (Mee, 2003).

Organizational factors are as important as individual attitudes in explaining nurses' behavior. "Geriatric nursing has suffered from the same problems as geriatric medicine: low prestige, poor pay, weak image" (Kane et al., 1981: 76). The paucity of geriatric nurses is also due to shortages within all areas of the profession, government regulations controlling what they do, and relatively poor salaries. Although few nursing schools provide extensive training in elder care, registered nurses resent competition from geriatric nurse practitioners because the latter tend to be less well trained but are remunerated as the market demands. Medicaid in some but not all states reimburses the services of physician's assistants and nurse practitioners, but Medicare covers only the work of nurses that is performed under a physician's supervision on-site. This latter regulation often limits the access of older people to primary care in rural areas. Finally, there is a matter of hygiene: a British study found that half of all nurses harbored an influenza infection, though they recalled suffering only a minor discomfort. Remaining at work meant that they potentially infected the very elderly patients, whom they meant to heal (British Geriatrics Society, 2001).

The same story applies to geriatric social workers, whose case load generally includes many elderly people. Social workers are trained to unravel thorny family issues and to circumvent bureaucratic legerdemain. Many find it easier to do their job if they view their older clients as dependent and treat them accordingly. For example, outpatient social workers at Massachusetts General Hospital were more likely to discuss a wider range of social and familial issues with younger than with older patients (Nelson, 2002: 352). Schools of social work have not been successful in teaching a positive image of age and aging. Institutions training social workers perpetuate ageism by offering few interdisciplinary gerontological courses in M.S.W. curricula (H. Johnson, 1995). When students are licensed, they tend to deny or limit services to elders because of institutional protocols in their work environment and bureaucratic red tape (Spicker et al., 1987: 29; Reed et al., 1992; B. Robinson, 1994).

Men and women over 65 consume more prescriptions and over-the-counter drugs than any other age group. The consumption of antidepressants and anti-anxiety drugs more than doubles and of hypnotic medications more than triples with advancing years (Grant, 1996; Pope, 2003). Older people are more likely to overuse medications or to continue taking drugs that their doctors no longer recommend. Despite widespread publicity about the pharmacological problems of elderly people, only 720 of the nation's 200,000 pharmacists have geriatric certification (Alliance for Aging Research, 2003: 3). They can hardly be expected to know how their aged customers take medications or if they are suffering because a drug has been withdrawn. Druggists' ignorance can have devastating effects: elderly patients have significantly higher adverse drug reactions than younger cohorts. Medicare recipients account for 1,900,000 adverse drug events a year; of these, 180,000 are life threatening or fatal. In some nursing homes, half of the resident population react poorly to drugs (Simon and Gurwitz, 2003; Tallis and Fillit, 2003: 1289–90). Pharmacists are not the only culprits; after all, it is physicians who prescribe medications. But gaps in the delivery of drugs powerfully underscore what happens when professionals are too busy to consult one another in sufficient detail as they try to offer older patients optimal care.

How Age Affects the Treatment of Acute Illnesses and the Care of Chronic Conditions

Biases learned in the course of professional training diminish the appeal of geriatrics among students. The negative ways in which many health-care practitioners choose to interact with older patients reduce the overall quality of care. Ageism also affects how professionals decide to treat specific acute illnesses and particular chronic conditions that large numbers of elderly patients present.

Heart disease is the leading cause of death among people over 65; it accounted for nearly half of the deaths of those over the age of 85 in 1991 (Hobbs and Damon, 1996: 3–9). Preventive measures clearly are warranted. Low doses of aspirin, for instance, cut by 25 percent the risk of a second heart attack or stroke. Elderly patients nonetheless are less likely than younger ones to receive beta-blockers, aspirin, and clot-dissolving drugs—medications known to reduce the likelihood of heart attacks (Health-Minder, 1999; Alliance for Aging Research, 2003: 8).

Furthermore, age is a deterrent in other ways. Surgeons cautiously select low-risk heart patients for procedures, for instance. Age variations in treatment are partly due to the fact that most people over 65 and virtually everyone over 75 (predominantly women) are excluded from clinical trials used to determine the effectiveness of various medications and procedures (Bowling, 1999). Researchers justify the age cut-off in recruiting patients for clinical trials in order to minimize complications due to co-morbidity. Transportation problems and preparing elderly people for tests, among other factors, make screening and testing burdensome, especially if it is presumed that including the aged population will not much affect outcomes. The omission of older recruits has expensive consequences: a 2003 study of Medicare beneficiaries who were hospitalized with chronic heart failure found that half the cases were preventable (Rich and Sox, 2000: 6; Alliance for Aging Research, 2003: 4–5).

In recent years there have been some signs that clinicians are responding to improvements in morbidity and mortality trends and deploying more preventive measures in treating heart disease. Directives have been issued for managing hypertension among the very old (Health Care Policy, 2004). Doctors are also beginning to prescribe statins, which have been proven to reduce the risk of ischemic heart disease by 30 percent among those over 75 by reducing high cholesterol. The value of this intervention would not have been evident through current trials, because statins are less effective in treating younger heart patients. That statins are generally efficacious (though they have been known to cause serious liver damage among the very old) is a point in favor of the future inclusion of more elders in clinical trials (T. Marshall, 2000: 1077; Alliance for Aging Research, 2003: 9).

Age biases also affect the treatment of cancer, the second leading cause of death among very old Americans. Epidemiologists have identified health behaviors, race and ethnicity, region of residence, and socioeconomic factors as influencing the likelihood of becoming a cancer victim (Shepherd, 1999). Age influences trends in diverse ways: between 1970 and 1990 there was a nearly 20 percent drop in the incidence of cancer among men and women between the ages of 45 and 54 compared to a 15 percent increase in cancer cases for men and 18 percent rise for women between the ages of 75 and 84. Some cancers decrease with advancing age: the incidence of breast cancer falls after age 85. The incidence of colorectal cancer, on the other hand, continues to rise among people entering their nineties. As in the case of heart disease, part of the age variation may be due to differences in treatment, notably if diagnoses are made at later stages of development, and the prevalence of comorbidities (Ciba, 1988: 175; Hobbs and Damon, 1996: 3–9; Institute of Medicine, 1999; Tallis and Fillit, 2003: 1297, 1305).

A University of Wisconsin study revealed that patients 75 and older were one-third less likely than younger patients to receive aggressive radiation treatment or chemotherapy. Older women with Stage III colon cancer, according to the *Archives of Surgery,* less frequently than younger women received chemotherapy. In a fifth of the latter cases, oncologists judged the patients to be too old for radiation; in a third of the cases, the physician simply did not offer the option. Similar patterns exist elsewhere in premier medical facilities. At Memorial Sloan-Kettering Cancer Center in New York, for instance, only 29 percent of the patients over 65 with ovarian cancer received aggressive treatment, compared to 63 percent of the younger ones (Alliance for Aging Research, 2003: 8). Roughly half the cases of breast cancer involve women over 65, but studies show that a smaller number of older women undergo mammography screening than younger women. Fewer breast-preservation surgeries and other appropriate therapies (such as chemotherapy) for breast cancer are performed on elderly women (Kent, 1999).

Experts do not recommend screening every older patient who may have cancer. The U.S. Preventive Services Task Force, for instance, ignored its own age cut-off in recommending that mammographies were warranted for women over 70 with prolonged exposure to estrogen and family histories of cancer. The same group considered prostate cancer screening, which nowadays is highly recommended by most clinicians for men over 50, to be "untenable" for those over 70 (Rich and Scott, 2000: 8, 9). Are the recommendations of the U.S. Preventive Services Task Force signaling a consensus about the overall efficacy of preventive measures in eldercare?

Increasingly, healthcare professionals seem to be recommending that patients over 65 receive the same cancer care as younger persons. Given the importance of early detection, screening and clinical trials should be made accessible to aged persons. Physicians should take into account the risk for the condition being investigated and the patient's expected chances for survival. Once cancer is detected, appropriate protocols should be followed. British oncologists report that the age of the patient does not serve per se as a robust predictor of complications or survival after surgery. Older patients remain under-represented in clinical trials, but they seem to respond as well to chemotherapy as do younger ones (Austin and Russell, 2003). After taking their patient's frailty and other conditions into account, doctors are increasingly being urged to screen men and women over 75. This subset of the elderly population on average has life expectancies sufficiently long to warrant intervention.

The way healthcare professionals treat cerebrovascular disease, the third leading cause of death among older Americans, conforms to the pattern in other domains. It is not so much that physicians invoke age per se in justifying treatments less complete and aggressive than they deliver to younger patients. Rather, they are inclined to cite other mitigating factors that they associate with old age, such as mental illness. For example, demented, elderly patients who have had a stroke are 2.5 times less likely to be prescribed aspirin or warfarin to prevent the risk of a second stroke (Manheimer, 1994: 429; American Geriatrics Society, 1998: 988–93). Denying an older demented person the treatment that a younger patient might expect as a matter of course could adversely affect the elder's potential quality of life.

Fear of the risks associated with frailty at advanced ages often affects surgeons' decisions about whether to operate. They worry that the intervention may do more harm than good. In so doing, they discount studies that justify surgery when necessary to save the lives of very old patients. A Mayo Foundation team of researchers reported that centenarians without a life-threatening disease could undergo surgery without increasing their immediate risk of death. Similarly, thanks to more available equipment and improved tolerance of dialysis, there has been a fourfold increase since 1996 in the number of patients over 74 who have started renal replacement therapy. In one study, more than 90 percent of the oldest patients had one or more co-morbid factors (mainly hypertension or heart disease). Among the indications, renal failure or a co-morbid condition accounted for early deaths; 38 percent died as a result of withdrawal from dialysis (Health-Minder, 1999; Munshi et al., 2001: 128–33).

Visits to the emergency room pose another set of dangers for older people. More than two-thirds of ER specialists lack geriatric training; they acknowledge that they feel less comfortable dealing with older patients than with younger adults. Nonetheless, in contrast to other doctors, emergency room specialists tend to shower elderly patients with services: older people are four times more likely than younger persons to avail themselves of ambulance services, five times more likely to be admitted to the hospital, and six times more likely to receive ER services. Not surprisingly, ER treatment comes at a high price. To this must be added the unpleasantness of the environment, the elderly patient's exclusion from trials of thrombolytic agents for myocardial infarctions, difficulties in transferring people from nursing home to the hospital and back, and the incidence of delirium—symptomatic of sepsis, drug toxicity, or some metabolic abnormality—among roughly a third of the patients discharged from emergency rooms (Sanders, n.d.).

Emergency room physicians rely on sophisticated equipment, the latest drugs, and high-tech monitoring to save lives. Older people, however, have to deal more with chronic conditions than acute accidents on a day-to-day basis; they typically can get by with access to low-level interventions. The recent emphasis on preventive medicine has been important in helping people maintain their vitality in later years. For instance, it is well documented that those who stop smoking at any age reduce their risk of heart attacks, chronic obstructive pulmonary diseases, and hearing loss. Quitting smoking after age 65 generally adds years to a life. But the success of preventive measures depends on getting the message across. Unfortunately, marketers and healthcare professionals often ignore or discount communicating the health benefits that might accrue to elderly patients if they decided to quit smoking.

"Older Americans are the forgotten victims of tobacco-related death and disease" according to the Center for Social Gerontology (1998: 1). Media researchers, service providers, and policymakers accord youth their top priority in their campaign to combat the tobacco industry's tempting promise that smoking is savvy and sexy. Obviously, it is imperative to dissuade teenagers from beginning to smoke. Nevertheless, it does not follow that efforts to persuade inveterate smokers to quit are useless. Marketers presume that those who have smoked for decades cannot quit. Some cynically reckon that long-term smokers will not live much longer anyway. Thus, little is said about older people, especially those with pulmonary problems, being vulnerable to second-hand smoke. Ageism plays a role here in editing older people out of the picture.

Elderly people are overlooked in other preventive care health campaigns as well. Some older people refuse to participate in alcohol rehabilitation programs. They deny their drinking problem and are rarely confronted about it (Gondolf, 1999: 10). Fitness clubs market to the young; YMCAs cater to youth and baby boomers. But appeals should be made to the older population as well because studies have documented that the initiation and maintenance of regular exercise of light to moderate intensity reduces the morbidity associated with chronic disease. Nonetheless, few scholars research the exercise habits of older adults; anecdotal evidence suggests that older patients with chronic disease are the most sedentary age group in the country (Petrella, 1999: 1, 8).

Similarly, changing the sexual habits and drug use of young adults has been a major focus in the campaign to prevent the spread of AIDS. Few programs, in contrast, have been targeted at mature adults. Data suggest that this is a mistake. Roughly 11 percent of all incidents of HIV occur in people over 50. The spread of AIDS has grown twice as fast in that age group as in younger age groups. Ageism is once again evident in discounting a population at risk. Older people are diagnosed later than younger victims, in part because fatigue, weight loss, and loss of memory are common to both the early stages of AIDS and to some pathways of senescence (Dixon, 2004).

Ageism also creates barriers to mental health care. Epidemiological studies document that more than a fifth of all Americans over 65 have a mental illness. These include Alzheimer's disease and neurodegenerative disorders, often accompanied by depression or psychosis. Mood disorders, bipolar illness, anxiety disorders, and severe illnesses such as schizophrenia and alcohol abuse are also prevalent in late life (S. Thompson,

1997; Streim, 2003: 1). Researchers contend that nearly two-thirds of all senior citizens with a mental disorder do not receive the treatment that they need. The proportion rises to 75 percent among those with depression. Although 65 to 80 percent of all nursing home residents have a diagnosable mental disorder, only a fifth receive care. Primary care physicians often fail to diagnose depression because they perceive the malady to be an "understandable" aspect of advancing years (Franz, 1999: 3; James, 2004). Knowing that no preventive intervention or health maintenance program has yet reduced the incidence of dementia among those over 85 justifies, in the minds of some doctors, their nihilistic posture.

Elderly people themselves are reluctant to step forward when they have a mental problem. Only 3 percent of those over 65 seek out mental and behavioral health professionals for assistance. Typically, they will present their mental health concerns, such as anxiety or somatization, as a physical malady when talking to their primary care physician (American Psychological Association, 2003b; APA, 2004). A 1990 study in Chicago found that a fifth of the cases of suicide investigated occurred within a day of a patient's visiting his or her primary care physician; 41 percent took their lives within a week, 84 percent within a month of the consultation. These data dramatically underscore the importance of early detection of mental illness among the aged population (Persky, 2004).

Despite the magnitude of the problem, most healthcare professionals express apathy and indifference toward the unmet mental health needs of older people. "If you look at the current infrastructure for meeting the needs of people over 65, it is as if mental illness doesn't exist for this population," says Franz (1999: 2). Links between primary care and social service, as well as between area agencies on aging and county mental health departments, are rarely coordinated. Disparities in Medicare and Medicaid reimbursements force social workers and psychologists to weigh the costs and benefits of dealing with elderly clients. Co-payments in general are higher for mental health treatment than for standard medical care, which deters those on fixed or low incomes to seek services. Given the concatenation of disincentives, ageism alone cannot be tagged as the prime cause for older people's lack of proper medical care, but it surely contributes to it.

The difficulties senior citizens face are often compounded by other factors in addition to, or besides, their advancing years. As we saw in chapter 1, women, African Americans, and other ethnic minorities tend to be sicker, poorer, and more isolated in their later years than older white men. Sexism and racism, like ageism, have institutional analogs to individual prejudices (Griffith, 2002). That said, the salience of ageism is noteworthy because of its interplay with independent factors. For example, in the strategic objectives for women's health care set forth in a 1995 U.N. Conference on Women, eight expansive paragraphs dealt with reproductive and sexual health, while only one terse paragraph focused on the needs of aging women (Kaveny, 1998). Ageism and sexism reinforce each other, but not always equally in complementary ways. In like manner does racism confound the effects of ageism and vice versa. Language barriers and cultural differences affect the care of elderly minorities, contributing to patient dissatisfaction. That said, epidemiologists would never claim on empirical grounds that they fully explain the higher incidence of chronic conditions such as asthma, obesity, and diabetes among older African Americans and Latinos than among Caucasians on the basis of age alone (Center on an Aging Society, 2004).

Finally, age discrimination may be hard to detect when researchers do not look for it. The amount of care Americans consume varies by the capacity of the health system where they live and the practices of doctors in that locality. But it is not clear that investigators who focus on geographical disparities in access to health care take fully into account variations in the relative proportion of old-old people in the area or age-related differences in mobility (Dartmouth Medical School, 1998; King's Fund, 2000). Sometimes, however, the connection between age and chronicity is palpable.

Consider the prevalence of ageism in long-term care centers, where 57 percent of the residents are over 65 and overwhelmingly women and dependent. To counterbalance a youth-oriented culture that loathes frailty, positive attitudes among health aides and nurses are essential in setting a salubrious tone. People who work in such facilities report that they are attracted by their positive experiences with older persons and their primary care responsibilities. Conversely, the negative image of long-term care articulated by the public and by their peers, poor pay, insufficient geriatric training, and lack of interest in old people are deterrents to attracting and retaining qualified healthcare personnel (National League for Nursing, 1988: 103–7; American Association of Homes and Services for the Aging, 2004).

The hierarchy of nursing homes, moreover, causes problems. Aides, not registered or practical nurses, do most of the hands-on care. Because of their proximity to the frail elderly, aides become the targets of residents' moodiness, fears, and anger. Add to this hard work, long hours, low wages and benefits, and roles stigmatized by society. These conditions are no mere figments of long-term care workers' imaginations. Poor working environments reinforce institutional ageism at a time when immigration rules diminish the potential pool of workers, and Medicare and Medicaid reimbursement policies restrict wages and benefits (Stone with Weiner, 2001: 3, 13; T. Nelson, 2002: 212–13). As a result, 10 to 40 percent of all nursing home residents receive inadequate care. Even disoriented residents understand what is going on. "Patients who feel they have been denied the right to choose their health plan . . . commonly go through a subjective experience analogous to those of being held captive" (Bursztajn and Brodsky, 1999; James, 2004).

End-of-life treatment raises the ethical, economic, and psychological stakes for healthcare practitioners and patients alike. Scientific professionals have for the most part moved beyond the position of equating old age with disease. But in an era of high technology, research breakthroughs, and wonder drugs, there is considerable controversy within both professional and lay circles concerning the relationship between aging and dying. Seven out of every ten deaths occur among people over 65; nearly a quarter of all deaths occur among those who are 85 or older (Hobbs and Damon, 1996: 3–4). Increases in health expenditures attributed to the extra years of a relatively healthy life are expected to be less than the costs concentrated at the end of life, where considerable Medicare outlays are expended (Yang et al., 2003). Defining death and facilitating dignified ways of dying become paramount, particularly against the backdrop of individual and institutional ageism that permeates the treatment of acute and chronic conditions.

Health officials in state health departments require a specific cause of death. The National Center for Health Statistics lists 113 cause-of-death classifications; "old age" is not among them (Rotstein, 2003). In only 5 percent of the forensic autopsy reports issued in Australia between 1988 and 1998 on 319 nonagenarians was no disease specified as the cause of death (HealthCentral, 2001). The prevailing expert opinion is that humans die of diseases and pathological disorders. However, some scientists point to other causes, such as wear and tear at the cellular level or genetic miscoding. For example, biogerontologist Leonard Hayflick, who demonstrated that cells reproduce fifty times before dying, believes that death probably results from accidents at the molecular level (1994: 235). Lengthening life from any of these perspectives increases the time span in which humans are subjected to fatal errors or illnesses beyond their control.

Other medical researchers contend that death is a "natural" phenomenon. "Life does have its natural, inherent limits," argues Sherwin Nuland in *How We Die* (1994: 70). "When those limits are reached, the taper of life, even in the absence of any specific disease or accident, simply sputters out." The basis for Nuland's opinion dates back to a treatise "On Youth and Old Age, On Life and Death, On Breathing," where Aristotle declaimed that "youth is the period of growth, . . . old age of its decay, while the intervening time is the prime of life." Dr. Nuland *would* list "old age" as the primary cause of a person's death.

Dubiety about the nature of death complicates decision making about the care of the dying. Some claim that "a *chance* of recovery is not a sufficient reason to embark on a treatment course if the chance is small, the hazards great, and the patient irreversibly demented" (Gillick, 1994: 41). Dr. Jerome Groopman, on the other hand, recommends giving patients choices by enabling them to understand their situation: "A treatment can have an unexpectedly dramatic impact. This is the great paradox of true hope: Because nothing is absolutely determined, there is not only reason to fear but also reason to hope" (2004: 210–11). Some ethicists opt for more pragmatic approaches. Daniel Callahan (1987) sparked considerable debate with his recommendation that age-specific treatment limits be set for withholding medical care. Critics excoriated Callahan's position as ageist. Nonetheless, some sort of rationing is inevitable. Choices must be made about the limits to be set. Many doctors prefer to assess the severity of co-morbid conditions instead of using age as a measure of predicting a patient's likely remaining time (Health and Age, 2004). Physicians are divided about the legal and ethical responsibility to withhold treatment to terminally ill patients, to use nasogastric feeding tubes, or to assist in suicide. Religiosity appears to be a key factor in how doctors react to these situations; significantly, the patient's age (or their own) is a less salient consideration (Quill, 1989b; MacKinnon et al., 2003).

Patients who lack advance directives or who have delegated medical powers of attorney rarely participate in the determinative process. Even those who have planned in advance may not see their wishes honored.

Older women are particularly vulnerable because many physicians do not communicate honestly with them about end-of-life options. Family members and friends at the bedside might distance themselves because their dying loved one reminds them of their own mortality (Carrese et al., 2002; T. Nelson, 2002: 50).

The unfolding dimensions of population aging will keep bioethicists at work for years to come. When Tithonos had finally outlived his virile youth and become a decrepit grasshopper, Greek mythology tells us, his lover Eos put him in a closet and threw away the key. This is not a viable option in the postmodern world. But the debate over an international policy for assisting the living dead has not yet begun. Pope John Paul II condemned euthanasia, even for those in a "vegetative state." Yet U.S. court decisions in the matter of two young women, Karen Ann Quinlan and Nancy Cruzan, indicate that this option remains open when there is no hope of regaining sentience.

Any attempt to reform the U.S. healthcare system to accommodate the needs and preferences of an aging population requires clear thinking. Choices are thorny at the individual, professional, and institutional levels. Age affects spending, but regulations concerning the distribution of resources and cost management are more important than demographics in increasing health expenditures (Getzen, 1992). The current bureaucratic thicket may require radical surgery.

A Proposal, at Once Modest and Grandiose, for Reform

By 2010, according to Senator John Breaux (2003b), "half of all doctors visits will be made by Americans over the age of 65. Despite this trend, America's healthcare system continues to engage in clear, consistent, age-based discrimination, preventing seniors from receiving healthcare services they need." Individual and institutionalized ageism thwarts meaningful reform. Eradicating age-based discrimination, or at least tempering its deleterious effects, must be the first order of business.

The Alliance for Aging Research (2003: 11–14) recommends four steps:

1. *Increase training and education of healthcare providers and research into aging.* The American Geriatrics Society, among other professional bodies, points to the shortage of geriatricians. It proposes financial incentives (such as reducing payment on loans and reimburs-

ing specialists for the extra time they spend with other clients) to d
more medical students into the specialty. The Alliance for Aging
Research supports such proposals, but it doubts that these measures
would suffice to make geriatrics as lucrative and prestigious as other
specialties.

Instead, the Alliance advises that every healthcare practitioner—
physician, nurse, social worker, psychologist, pharmacist, and allied
health professional—receive intensive training in caring for elderly
patients as part of the curriculum. To this should be added the idea
of professional training around evidence-based practices to promote
exposure to healthy as well as impaired elders (Hodkinson, 1975: 150;
Tonks, 1999; President's New Freedom Commission on Mental
Health, 2002: 3). Several groups recommend the addition of geriatric
competency in licensing and credentialing examinations. And they
urge the federal government and philanthropies to invest more money
into the generation and dissemination of basic research so that more
progress can be made in understanding the processes of aging and of
curing or treating diseases prevalent in late life.

2. *Include older patients in clinical trials.* Medicare, in the Alliance's opinion, should encourage the involvement of elderly people in
new drug trials as well as in treatments for heart disease and cancer
to identify potential problems besetting the oldest old (see also R. Butler, 2003). Community groups and advocates for elderly people
should publicize the importance of such clinical trials and take steps
to facilitate older people's participation. Similarly, greater emphasis
should be placed on optimizing the use of automation in promoting
the independence of elderly people. Low-cost passive technologies,
such as sleep monitors and motion sensors, effectively check on activities before a crisis occurs (Alliance for Aging Research, 2004: 15–18).

3. *Use appropriate screening and treatment methods.* Although
Medicare covers some screening, older people do not have access to
other tests. Excluding elderly people is counterproductive because
early detection and prevention usually facilitates treatment. To accomplish this goal, the Alliance envisions an ambitious educational
program. Patients and their families need to understand the importance of screening. As is the case with clinical trials, physicians' fears
concerning untoward risks in subjecting older people to screening
must be allayed.

4. *Empower and educate older Americans.* Efforts must be made

to persuade older people to become more proactive in preventing disease, in questioning their physicians and care providers, and in describing aches and pains instead of attributing them to old age. Older patients can make doctors better if first-year residents are given time enough to take lengthy interviews that reveal the total person (Kleinfeld, 2004b). Although the baby boom generation has a reputation for being outspoken, it is not clear that their earlier political activism will translate into a posture of aggressive management when they confront their healthcare needs.

The recommendations proposed by the Alliance for Aging Research resonate with those made by other organizations, but they do not exhaust the list of incremental steps that might be taken to reform elder care. For instance, multidisciplinary geriatric assessment teams might be more effectively used. The value of this approach was demonstrated in the mid-1980s in a randomized control trial that resulted in reduced mortality rates, more accurate diagnoses, and fewer nursing home placements (Mezey et al., 2002: 30).

Best-practice models exist. Perhaps the best known is the On Lok program in San Francisco. Originally an adult day care center, On Lok was a pioneer in providing acute care and long-term services to the heretofore underserved predominantly minority, low-income, functionally impaired population. The On Lok model has been replicated across the country in Programs of All-Inclusive Care for the Elderly (PACE). Another model program, the Georgia Source Program, links acute and long-term care by using Medicaid's concept of primary care case management. Also worth noting is the Jewish Home and Hospital Lifecare System, which serves 5,200 older adults daily at three locations in metropolitan New York. Fourth-year Mount Sinai Medical School students have a mandatory rotation through the system. Former First Lady Rosalynn Carter has established an Institute for Caregiving to promote greater effectiveness among professional and family caregivers across the life span. And the Cambridge (Mass.) Health Alliance has convened a "council of elders" to serve as senior mentors in teaching medical residents and nursing students how to deal with older patients (Suchman et al., 2000; Mezey et al., 2002: 190; Jewish Home and Hospital Lifecare System, 2004; Carter, 2004; Alliance for Aging Research, 2004: 7–8).

Another valuable but independent type of network would inform citizens about age-related healthcare policy developments at the local, state, and national levels. Interest groups such as AARP and the National Council on Aging have elaborate Web sites that discuss changes in licensure, personnel training, and insurance coverage. It is critical that geriatric educators be involved and internships be offered to students who wish to focus on the needs of older people (Health Resources and Services Administration, 2004). It is especially important to monitor developments in Washington, because Congress ultimately has the greatest leverage, legislatively and fiscally, to make things change.

Because it is impossible to survey all the areas in which the federal government affects the delivery of health care to older Americans, let me focus on one area that needs rethinking: research on societal aging. The National Institute on Aging, the Administration on Aging, the Department of Veterans Affairs, and the Social Security Administration generate more research than any university-based center or think tank. The Public Health Service's Agency for Healthcare Research and Quality has a mandate to support basic research and demonstration grants "to demonstrate how the health care system can most cost-effectively prevent disability, reduce functional decline, and extend active life expectancy in older people" (2001: 5). Yet these agencies typically overlook the significance of population aging.

One example will suffice. In 1995 the Department of Health and Human Services embarked on a five-year project to produce *Healthy People 2010.* Organizers consulted federal and state mental health, substance abuse, and environmental agencies. They convened focus groups and forged partnerships. Works-in-progress were made public for review and comment. The result was a two-volume compendium with data focusing on twenty-eight areas, ranging from medical product safety, to immunization, to maternal, infant, and child health. Incredibly, in the face of population aging and the graying of the baby boom cohort, the compilers paid scant attention to late-life issues. "Age is not included in the minimum table because showing inclusive age categories would add considerable complexity to the minimum set," said *Healthy People 2010* (U.S. Dept. of Health and Human Services, 2000: RG-7). There are eighteen references to the "elderly" in the index, but none to "longevity," "life expectancy," or "population aging." That no compendium can be encyclopedic does not obviate the need to pay attention to age and aging.

In the face of such myopia, it is tempting to end on a radical note.

Incremental steps, long the staple of U.S. policy-making, are not enough. Consider the length of time it took to enact the flawed Prescription Drug Improvement and Modernization Act of 2003 as Medicare Part D, despite the fact that fewer retirees get drug coverage from their employers (Abelson, 2003). Moreover, few see any hope of restoring the 1988 Medicare Catastrophic Coverage Act, which was doomed when wealthy senior citizens realized that they would be financing the initiative (Palmore, 1999: 144). Efforts to modernize Medicare by merging Parts A and B do not seem worth the effort because the savings and added coverage would be trivial. Other proposals to restructure Medicare overlook the provisions that baby boomers will require (American Association of Homes and Services for the Aging, 2002; Moon, 2001). Fundamental reforms are necessary to meet the healthcare needs of an aging population. Let me propose three.

First, the moment seems propitious to reconsider *national health insurance*. Denounced throughout the twentieth century as a Socialist-inspired, expensive, inefficient way of delivering care, national health insurance has attracted the support of an unlikely array of groups. For the first time in its history, the Institute of Medicine has urged the adoption of national health insurance by 2010, primarily to extend protection to millions of uninsured Americans ("Science Panel Urges Universal US Health Insurance," 2004). Nine thousand doctors, including two former U.S. Surgeons General, a former editor of the *New England Journal of Medicine,* and a number of medical school professors have formed Physicians for a National Health Program. Their plan promises universal, comprehensive coverage; it gives patients free choice in selecting doctors and hospitals (J. Chapman, 2003; Nader, 2003). Also supporting the concept are the League of Women Voters and the Catholic Health Association of the United States (Place, 2000; League of Women Voters, 2003). Stuart Butler, a senior official at the conservative Heritage Foundation, decries the current "patchwork of public and private programs with widely differing eligibility criteria." The nation's employment-based health systems, in his opinion, can lay the groundwork for universal coverage, but Congress would have to enunciate and underwrite the goals (S. Butler, 2003).

There are several ways to design a national health insurance system for the United States. The most popular proposal is a "single tax-funded comprehensive insurer in each state, federally mandated but locally controlled" (Woolhandler and Himmelstein, 2002). Savings from current administrative costs, which total 30 percent of present expenditures, would pay for expanded coverage. Because variations on a single-payer system have featured prominently in past reform debates, this option will face considerable political opposition from critics with well-honed arguments. Karen Davis, president of the Commonwealth Fund, urges that the federal government use its clout to negotiate more aggressively for limiting the costs of medical services instead of relying on third parties (such as insurance companies) to determine market prices. Davis would combine all group insurance options, ranging from employer-based plans, federal employee programs, plans for small businesses and individuals, and provisions for people with low incomes (K. Davis, 2004: 8, 16). A third option builds on another recommendation made by Davis. The "pincer strategy" eschews a single-payer model. Instead, it would incrementally extend Medicare eligibility down to age 55, to reach a vulnerable segment of the population—older adults out of work and disabled persons waiting to become eligible for insurance coverage (Oberlander and Marmor, 2002). I would propose expanding Medicare— because it is more popular (63% like it) than private health plans (19%) (Randall, 2003: 5)—to cover the institutional costs of chronic conditions, and let Medigap insurance fill the cracks.

In each plan, the needs of an aging population are met better than presently. Medical health coverage would be transgenerational and affordable—though more expensive to citizens. Each idea pays attention to the chronic long-term care needs of older adults, providing coverage for preventive medicine, screening, and clinical trials. And each aims to educate older people about how to select the care they require.

Second, the United States should embark on a *reform of medical education* to accommodate the needs of an aging population. The impact should be comparable to the changes implemented as a result of the Flexner Report a century ago. Currently, specialists dominate the nation's healthcare system. Most of the best-known physicians specialize in a subspecialty; for their expertise and efforts (super)specialists enjoy fascinating intellectual challenges and creative problem-solving, not to mention handsome salaries and considerable prestige.

Yet most Americans present ailments that do not really require the services of specialists. Well-trained general practitioners and nurses could deal sufficiently with most people's physical complaints. According to one study (Radin and Achenbaum, forthcoming), roughly 70 percent of all patients make a doctor's appointment for what might be considered a straightforward purpose—an annual physical is the primary reason. They want relief from colds and flu. They seek pre- and postnatal care. They present high blood pressure, angina, acute sprains and strains, pneumonia, ear infections, skin rashes, acne, and sinus problems, to mention the most common. Clearly, referrals to specialists would be necessary for cancers, many mental illnesses, displaced fractures, and other severe emergencies.

Relying more heavily on well-trained general practitioners for eldercare would be a boon to older adults. States with more specialists who deal with the elderly experience higher costs and lower quality of care (Baicker and Chandra, 2004). More family practice physicians, psychiatrists, and internists should be certified in geriatrics. The chronic conditions that bedevil senior citizens generally are debilitating and painful if left untreated, but primary care physicians with sufficient education and experience should be able to make proper diagnoses, prescribe appropriate medications, and recommend an efficacious course of treatment. Similarly, general practitioners and nurses can acquire the training necessary to detect acute maladies early on, though there is no hard evidence of a relationship between nurses and high-quality care (ibid.: 193). More philanthropies should follow the lead of the John A. Hartford Foundation in expanding the training of doctors, nurses, social workers, and other health professionals as they integrate the delivery of services for older adults (JAHF, 2005).

Ideally, we need a 50–50 mix of generalists and specialists. To achieve this goal, we probably should establish two types of medical schools. One would resemble institutions such as Johns Hopkins and Harvard: they would train specialists who would do biomedical research. The latter sort of institutions would produce practitioners-of-first-contact, dedicated to community-based service. This proposal is bound to be criticized on several fronts. Aspiring medical students would resist being guided into careers in areas that traditionally have paid less and afforded less prestige than specialties. Americans, accustomed to the very best, might feel "cheated" if they could not be seen by a well-known expert. But the nation's over-reliance on specialization costs a lot of money. Patients need to be educated that their maladies, while deserving competent attention, may not be as exotic or unique as they presume. At the very least, they must understand that their co-pays do not begin to cover the cost of visiting a specialist.

This leads, third, to ways to *make older and younger patients more astute consumers of medical care.* There is no free lunch, so the saying goes, but it is a well-documented fact that when third parties pick up a substantial part of the tab for medical care, people are inclined to use more services than if they have to pay directly. With cost containment a priority, the current third-party system means few choices are available at high rates. Like physicians, informed older people complain about the increasing welter of state laws and reimbursement regulations that restrict their access to healthcare services, including nontraditional treatments such as acupuncture and massage therapy. Conversely, government-mandated benefit services tend to increase insurance costs, causing some individuals and companies (especially small firms) to drop their coverage, which then increases the number of uninsured Americans (Blevins, 1997: 2–3).

Over the past two decades, in an effort to cut costs, more and more firms have been reconsidering what percentage of their employees' health benefits they should pay. Between 1980 and 1993, the proportion of employers who provided comprehensive health benefits fell from 74 to 37 percent. Now, employers are inclined to deny health benefits to part-time workers. This decision especially affects the coverage of women and minorities. The decline in employment-based health benefits is exacerbated by the shift from a manufacturing to a service economy in the United States (Strom, 2003; Fronstin, 2004). Some health economists think that making individuals pay their own costs would add efficiency to the system. Others note that shifting the full cost to patients will put a burden on older employees who will not be able to afford higher premiums and out-of-pocket expenses (Johnson, 2002).

Several compromise options exist. The Bush administration prefers vouchers, but that approach would not help low-income recipients any more than vouchers help the poor in the educational sphere. Furthermore, vouchers could be expected to drive up costs, as consumers demanded more generous vouchers to offset higher insurance costs. A number of economists have suggested refundable, prepayable tax credits up to 50 percent of the premium. Some think the credits should go directly to individuals, possibly adjusted according to age group (Blevins, 1997: 10–11; Frogue, 2001). Others suggest that a "franchiser" is necessary to assist the vulnerable elderly, among others, and to monitor outcomes (Bowman, 2001; Woolhandler and Himmelstein, 2002). Under all of these scenarios, private insurance companies will play a less prominent role than they do now, but they are likely to remain part of any reconfiguration. Underwriters would continue doing assessments, and companies like Wells Fargo Elder Services, which integrate their clients' health care and financial services, would serve as models for helping older people determine their priorities in order to remain at home.

These "grandiose" closing recommendations have deliberately been left sketchy so as not to detract from the point of origin for any meaningful reform. The extent and virulence of ageism in the U.S. healthcare system exceeds that found in the marketplace or educational institutions. The prejudice against age among all participants is deep. Despite improvements in the health of senior citizens, gains in life expectancy, and public awareness of the likely impact of the baby boom generation on healthcare costs, we persist in the negative, nihilistic attitudes and practices that characterized the American way of medicine thirty years ago (Breaux, 2003a). Until our perspectives on aging and dying catch up with the realities of prolonged senescence, the resilience and constraints that come with extra years, we are doomed to tinker with minutia instead of facing the real challenges and opportunities that lie ahead.

Renewing Religious Experiences and Spiritual Practices for a New Age } 5

"The religious atmosphere of the country was the first thing that struck me on arrival in the United States," observed Alexis de Tocqueville in *Democracy in America*. "In France I had seen the spirits of religion and freedom almost always marching in opposite directions. In America, I found them intimately linked together in joint reign over the same land" (1836b: 295). The French nobleman supposed that some Americans acted religiously out of habit rather than conviction, their professions of belief tinged with a certain degree of hypocrisy. Still, de Tocqueville's critique of the pervasiveness and novelty of America's "religious atmosphere" was well grounded. His visit occurred after the creation of the American Bible Society (1816), the American Sunday School Union (1824), and the American Home Missionary Society (1826). De Tocqueville's trip coincided with the fervent preaching of Charles Grandison Finney and his "Holy Band" of co-workers in urban centers. On the frontier were evangelical preachers "hawking the word of God from place to place" (ibid.: 535; for context, see Rozwenc and Bender, 1978: 1:435–36). "Whole families, old men, women and children cross difficult country and make their way through untamed forests to come great distances to hear [the revivalists]," de Tocqueville wrote. "When they arrive and listen to them, for several days and nights they neglect to look after their affairs and even forget the most pressing needs of the body. Here and there throughout American society you meet men filled with an enthusiastic, almost fierce spirituality such as cannot be found in Europe. From time to time strange sects arise which strive to open extraordinary roads to eternal happiness" (1836b: 535).

The United States, unlike most European nations, had no established church. Observances here were less ritualized. Despite the number of competing sects and denominations, people in the new world, de Tocqueville claimed, "all see their religion in the same light. . . . America is still the place where the Christian religion has the greatest real power over men's souls" (ibid.: 449, 291).

American Religious Pluralism Becomes Eclectic and Cosmopolitan

If self-reported survey data in this domain can be trusted (for reservations on whether Americans exaggerate their practices, see B. A. Robinson, 2001: 2; Adherents.com, 2002: 5), the United States remains one of the most fervently religious nations in the world. According to a 1991 International Social Survey, only Filipinos and Poles exceed the percentage of Americans who express no doubt about the existence of God; U.S. adults are more inclined than respondents elsewhere to affirm life after death, the devil, hell, and religious miracles; the Irish barely surpass the proportion of Americans who believe in heaven (Bishop, 1999: 7–10). Deeds speak. William James asserted in *The Varieties of Religious Experience* that "prayer is religion in act; that is, prayer is real religion" (1902: 454). Piety by this measure is ubiquitous in the United States, for Americans—at least 85 percent surveyed in every demographic category—pray more often than they go to church. More than three-quarters pray at least once a week; over half, daily. Even a fifth of those who characterize themselves as atheists or agnostics claim to pray daily (Fagan, 1996: 1).

Religious affiliation is difficult to measure in the United States because of the number, size, and diverse structures of faith communities. In 2001, 81 percent of the adult population identified with a religious body, down 9 percent from 1990 (Kosmin et al., 2001: 10). Mainstream institutions have lost ground: the percentage of Americans claiming to be Christian fell from 86 percent to 77 percent between 1990 and 2001. Although the Roman Catholic Church is the largest social institution in the United States, a quarter to a third of its membership does not belong to a parish;

only 5 percent of adults under thirty attend Mass (Leege and Trozzolo, n.d.: 4–5). The expansion of the Southern Baptist Convention has not kept pace with the nation's population growth, though American Baptist churches have grown in the west since 1997. Membership in the Episcopal and Presbyterian churches, among other prominent Protestant denominations, actually declined (Cho, 2002; Breen, 2003). There is a shortage of ordained leadership in many religious communities. The Roman Catholic Church is consolidating parishes and relying on women to give religious instruction and promote spiritual growth as its number of priests shrinks. Some Protestant churches face a dwindling pool of clergy, many of whom they cannot afford to pay full-time (Leege and Trozzolo, n.d.: 14; Waken, 2003: 26; *Courier-Journal,* 2004).

A different picture of religion in America emerges, however, if we extend our field of vision. Harvard anthropologist of religion Diana Eck claims that "'We the people' of the United States now form the most profusely religious nation on earth" (quoted in Kosmin et al., 2001: 5). The number of congregations in the United States is estimated to range from 200,000 to 450,000. Roughly half of these communities have from 100 to 400 members. Researchers count 200 to 1,600 denominations in America, representing all the world religions (Tirrito and Cascio, 2003: 32–35). Some sects and denominations are geographically limited: only the Roman Catholic and United Methodist churches have congregations in all fifty states (Adherents.com, 2002a: 19). As de Tocqueville noted long ago, Americans tend to join and leave faith communities as their family circumstances and personal needs change.

The chief beneficiaries of this propensity to shift affiliations have been evangelical and fundamentalist groups. Evangelical/born-again and Pentecostal assemblies, for instance, experienced gains of 42 percent and 16 percent, respectively, between 1990 and 2001. Nondenominational churches grew 37 percent during the same period (Kosmin et al., 2001: 24; Craemer, 2003; Stern, 2003). Born-again Christians are more inclined than the average American churchgoer to claim that their religious beliefs have changed their behavior. Two-thirds of all evangelicals report that they read the Bible during the past week compared to two-fifths of those attending mainline congregations who were surveyed about their religious practices (B. A. Robinson, 2001: 2). Nearly two-thirds of all Americans with access to a computer used the Internet for spiritual or religious purposes (Tirrito and Cascio, 2003: 31; Pew, 2004).

Religious observances and practices vary by demographic subsets. Thanks to the influx of people from Mexico and other Latin American countries, the proportion of Latinos who consider themselves Catholic has remained constant since the late 1980s. The percentage drops, however, from 74 percent among first-generation immigrants, to 72 percent among the second generation, to 62 percent among the third. The proportion of Protestant Latinos, conversely, rises from 15 percent among the oldest generation to 29 percent among the youngest. There are more Latino Protestants in the United States than Jews, Muslims, Episcopalians, and Presbyterians combined (Espinosa et al., 2003: 14–17; Kosmin et al, 2001: 8). Twelve percent of the Hispanic population indicate that they practice no religion. Due to proselytism by the Catholic Charismatic movement and the growth of Pentecostalism, however, more than a quarter of all Latinos (and 85 percent of Latino Protestants) claim to be born-again or spirit-filled. Lay leadership opportunities, healing ministries, and greater liturgical roles for women account for the appeal. Moreover, at both ends of the spectrum—from liberation theology to fundamentalist religiosity—there is an impetus for adherents to insist that religion engage in social, economic, and educational reform. Three-quarters of all Latinos want religious organizations to aid undocumented immigrants even if it means breaking the law; three-fifths believe that illegal aliens should be eligible for welfare and Medicaid.

Religious practices vary by age as well as ethnicity. Not only does the baby boomer generation "shop" for suitable congregations among established denominations, but they have also been receptive to incorporating traditions from Eastern sources into their religious practice. Buddhism has arrived on Main Street, appealing alike to Caucasians, African Americans, Latinos, and Asians who reconvert. Boomers incorporate the mantra of Buddha, which connects wisdom and compassion with action, into their devotions and daily lives. "Today, Christian thinkers can count Buddhist ideas and practices among the building blocks from which they may construct theologies and spiritual exercises" (Arthur, 2004: 8; see also Della Santina, 1989; Nattier, 1997). Aspects of Islam syncretize American religiosity. Should current trends persist, Islam will be the second largest religion in the United States after Christianity by 2015. Many blacks join the Islamic community to affirm their pan-African identity. Muslim membership grows as its charities reach out to the urban poor (Webb, 1995; Haddad, 1991).

Other links to multifaith religious sites have proliferated in recent decades. At one extreme, religious seekers practice Wicca and witchcraft; others conjure with Druids and Norse-Pagans (Fairgrove, 1994). To satisfy people's hunger for something different, establishment institutions adapt their religious education programs. St. Bartholomew's Church on New York City's Park Avenue hired a rabbi to direct its Center for Religious Inquiry. In spring 2004, it offered a Pre-Passover Seder, conversations between the parish's rector and the center director, and courses with topics ranging from Sufism, Hinduism, biomedical ethics, Mary Magdalene, Ann Frank, Christian atonement, the monks of Tibhirine, and aging (St. Bartholomew's, 2004).

This eclectic, cosmopolitan approach is bound to alter the context of religious experiences in late life. Throughout U.S. history, a greater proportion of older people than any other age group has considered themselves religious. According to the 2001 American Religious Identification Survey (Kosmin et al., 2001: 21, 31–32), four-fifths of those over age 65 acknowledged a religious outlook on life compared to roughly two-thirds of those between 18 and 34. Senior citizens constitute about a third of most mainline Protestant denominations—three times as many congregants are over the age of 65 than under 35. (Buddhism and Islam claim the highest proportion of youth members in the United States.) More than half of the affiliated elderly attend their place of worship every week. These regular members are inclined to trust their clergy's guidance. They also volunteer their time and energy within the congregation as well as serving youth, children, and families in the community who are nonmembers (Tirrito and Cascio, 2003: 41, 145, 173–74).

U.S. synagogues and churches, adhering to Hebrew Scripture and New Testament injunctions, have traditionally offered social services and housing for their elderly. In the late nineteenth century, for instance, Americans built old-age homes for specific ethnic groups within the Roman Catholic Church and other denominations (Achenbaum, 1978a: 82). Three-fifths of all Catholic parishes now have some organized ministry for aged people. Larger jurisdictions, such as the Diocese of Pittsburgh (2004), offer respite care, information and referral, outreach training, intergenerational programs, and educational opportunities to serve and enrich late life. Catholic Charities USA provides training, technical assistance, and opportunities via the Internet to work with the aging (2002).

Protestants follow suit. The Adventist Development and Relief Agency, incorporated in 1956, now runs 9 regional and 120 local offices throughout the country to coordinate service projects and relief efforts (2003). A 1987 American Baptist Resolution on Older Americans insists that older people serve as well as be served. Elderly people are to "be change agents in the events and affairs of church and society." Baptist seminaries and institutions of higher learning sensitize students to work with and on behalf of elderly people, forming educational and social partnerships between congregations and long-term care facilities. Clergy and lay leaders empower elderly people to promote their self-sufficiency (American Baptist Church, 1987). Episcopal Senior Ministries in the Diocese of Washington, D.C., has sponsored volunteer services and worked with grassroots organizations and national associations since 1924 to sponsor assisted living, transportation, and caregiving (Episcopal Senior Ministries, 2004).

Community-based Jewish social service agencies and nursing homes typically set the standard for eldercare. Larger Jewish federations are also pacesetters. Since 1936 the B'nai B'rith International has had three priorities: the aged, youth, and advocacy for Jewry worldwide. For the first time in 2001, twenty-three leading Jewish advocacy groups, service providers, and religious organizations formed the Jewish Coalition for Long Term Care, particularly to advance wellness programs and to find solutions for the chronic shortage of healthcare providers (American Jewish Communities, 2001; B'nai B'rith International, 2002; Holtz, 2003). Jewish community service agencies report a positive association between work and well-being among senior adult workers (Stevens-Roseman, 2004).

Mindful of the growth and increasing diversity of their older congregants, clergy and lay leaders are trying new approaches to reach their aging flocks. Unlike most medical schools, seminaries have made it a priority to teach young ministers how to relate to senior citizens (Fuchs, 2003). The Roman Catholic Church established Holy Apostles College and Seminary in Connecticut to train older men for the clergy (Praize, 2004). Episcopal Senior Ministries (2002) conducted a survey to identify variations in health care, housing, and caregiving needs among African Americans, gays, and Hispanics over 50 in the Diocese of Washington. The Episcopal Diocese of Albany in 2003 established CEDAR (The Christian Elder Dispositions, Arbitrations and Reconciliation Court), an interdenominational venue that helps homeowners and contractors and other people settle their dispute out of court (*Living Church,* 2003: 34). In 2000 the American Baptist Church launched "Rekindle!" which relies on video conferencing technology to enable church elders to exchange ideas about renewing their congregations (Stanford, 2001).

Nondenominational bodies sometimes transform traditional concepts into fresh action plans. Interfaith Ministries, for instance, works with churches and synagogues to train volunteer caregivers. In Houston, Interfaith Ministries serves as a conduit to the Foster Grandparent Program (Interfaith Ministries, 2004; HCR Manor Care, 2003: 3). Because American Indians value the wisdom associated with age, some Native American reservations have taken steps to invest older men and women with additional authority. An Elders Leadership Training Camp instructs older people on how to define and redirect religious priorities. Its proponents hope that it will give the necessary "training, encouragement, and spiritual endowment . . . to see revival and people's hearts won to God" (John, 2004: 21; Elders Camp, 2004; Wall, 1993). Meanwhile, other service agencies continue assisting elderly people as they know best. The Salvation Army, for example, operates 509 residential centers caring for nearly 9,000 senior residents in 107 countries.

Ethnic groups have transplanted traditional values to the United States. In Korean households and churches, where filial piety flourishes, considerable attention is given to services to and activities for elderly people. Pastors set the tone, mobilizing the community. Lacking the wherewithal to hire trained personnel, paraprofessionals run service programs. Members of virtually every congregation make pastoral visits to the homebound; most encourage their older members to play an active role in liturgies and outreach programs. Nor do Koreans insulate themselves. In Los Angeles, the Hebron Presbyterian Church, located in an African-American neighborhood, donated Korean food to local residents one Thanksgiving. Thereafter, Korean and African-American church leaders sponsored social events. Then came joint services and choir exchanges, culminating in 1991 in the African/Korean Christian Alliance. This partnership reduced tensions during the riots in Los Angeles a year later and became a model for alliances in New York, Chicago, and other cities (Tirrito and Cascio, 2003: 162–67).

The number and range of religious-based programs for aged people look (deceptively) impressive. To fulfill their charters, *all* congregations offer social service activities to members; nearly three-fifths provide clothes, food, or shelter for individuals in their neighborhood, engage in community development, and are involved in organizing redevelopment ventures. But most outreach is performed by large, wealthy congregations with a sense of mission. Small churches must rely on fewer staff, already burdened with too many commitments, to muster time and energy for civic purposes: only one in twenty of all U.S. congregations has designated at least one staff person for outreach development. Even the direct support for community building delivered by median-sized congregations represents a modest 3 percent of their budget (Dionne and Chen, 2001: 10–11, 288).

Because approximately three-fifths of the public thinks that President George W. Bush's reliance on religion in policy-making is appropriate, it is not surprising that many endorse his contention that "government can and should support social services provided by religious people, as long as those services go to anyone in need, regardless of their faith. And when government gives that support, charities and faith-based programs should not be forced to change their character or compromise their mission" (Pew Forum on Religious and Public Life, 2003: 2–3; Bush, 2002: i). The Reverend Leon Sullivan, through his Zion Baptist Church in Philadelphia, established a prototype in the early 1960s for community development corporations supported by public and private funds. Elderly blacks, especially those from African and African-Caribbean cultures, have been prime movers for faith-based initiatives because they want to acculturate the young and reduce crime (Ritts, 2000; Reddie, 2001). Lutheran Social Services, Catholic Charities, the Jewish Federation, and the Salvation Army, among others, forged federal partnerships long before current laws facilitated support.

The religious community, as de Tocqueville noted, "restricts itself to its own resources . . . [but there are] important political consequences resulting from this novel situation" (1836c: 299, 295). Faith-based organizations have discussed with the Bush administration ways to enhance the ethics of long-term care (Rosenthal, 2001). Twice as many older Americans—about half of those surveyed—say that they would be more comfortable with volunteer help from a faith-based organization than from a secular institution (Intrados, 2003: 4–5). College-aged people and teens are more enthusiastic about faith-based initiatives than their elders (Gilmore, 2002). Support divides along racial lines: nearly two-thirds of African-American congregations express an interest in applying for federal funds, compared to only a quarter of white congregations (Dionne and Chen, 2001: 11). Wealthy black churches in impoverished neighborhoods that are led by dynamic clergy, and congregations in poor neighborhoods composed of (lower) middle-class members of any race who are committed to social change, view faith-based programs as ways to achieve social justice while energizing the membership: "The religious will encounter the secular . . . the sacred will encounter the civic" (ibid.: 15).

Religion and Healthful Aging

The eclectic, cosmopolitan patterns woven into American religious pluralism represent one of the distinguishing features of contemporary faith communities. The connection between religion and healthful aging is a second hallmark—in this instance linking soul and body, mystery and science. A note of caution must be sounded before reviewing the literature. Many medical practitioners consider the empirical relationship between religious observances and good health in late life to be weak and inconsistent. Some dismiss all alternative approaches to healing as New Age quackery, placebos at best. To persuade skeptics and enthusiasts alike, more controlled studies generating hard data are necessary (Julian, 2001; Chippendale, 2004; Larson, 1993: 50).

Proponents of the efficacy of belief and prayer in the care and treatment of patients are careful in reporting results. They write in terms of correlational factors, not causal relationships. They, too, worry about the quality of research designs and the application of blind controls, lest spurious science raise false expectations. Still, investigators into the "biology of belief" and "the healing power of faith" are attracting attention in medical circles; their books sell well (Benson, 1997; Koenig, 1999). And it is significant that the National Institutes of Health began in 1990 to fund research on religion and aging; five years later it convened experts to map out a national plan for research and clinical practice in this area of alternative medicine. Both the scientific community and religious congregations are beginning to take seriously the heretofore undervalued role of prayer and faith in promoting healthful longevity.

Systematic sociological research into the association between religion and mortality actually began at least a century ago. In *Suicide* (1897),

Emile Durkheim theorized and documented that religious people were less likely to take their own lives than secular men and women. Case studies of Mormons and Seventh Day Adventists during the second third of the twentieth century indicated that strict adherents of these groups had lower mortality risks than individuals with casual or no allegiance to a faith community. Initial and subsequent analyses of the longitudinal data generated by the Alameda County (California) Study and Tecumseh (Michigan) Community Health Study indicated that church membership contributed to the value of good health practices, stable marriages, and strong social contacts in lowering the risk of premature death (Koenig and Cohen, 2002: 264–65). Subsequent investigations have refined these pioneering studies.

In the current wave of work, researchers have focused on mental health issues in late life. Religious resources that bolster a person's sense of identity and authenticity, investigators reported, serve as coping mechanisms. In some instances, they noted, religious obsessions might induce guilt, thereby complicating the course of recovery. In the mid-1970s a new field, psychoneuroimmunology, was developed to study the interrelationships among the nervous, endocrine, and immune systems on mental and physical health. Since then, a number of studies have documented an association between religion and the immune function. Mounting research makes it reasonable to hypothesize that, when individuals invoke their faith, they activate areas of their brains that in turn inhibit stress responses (Koenig and Cohen, 2002: viii, 31). For instance, Dr. Harold Koenig and colleagues tracked the rates of depression in 161 men under 40 and 850 men over 65 admitted between 1987 and 1989 to the Durham, North Carolina, VA hospital. The research team measured self-assessments and observer-rated symptoms and used a battery of tests to evaluate depressive disorders cross-sectionally and longitudinally. "Religious coping either relieved depression or prevented it from occurring," they concluded (Koenig, 1994: 227; see also 144, 222–23; Koenig and Lawson, 2004).

Several churches in the 1970s and 1980s independently reported successful outcomes in launching programs to raise awareness about mental health and to support congregants suffering from depression and other mental illnesses (Fallot, 1988: 36–37, 69–71). Scientific data lent credence to these initiatives. Belief in God and social support (with some exceptions), report investigators, prevent responses to stressful events that are harmful to health by increasing people's perception that they can cope with stressful situations. "Religious groups may be more effective at providing these benefits than other domains and they may facilitate access to other social domains as well. However, the relative efficacy of religious participation in affecting health is not yet established" according to Koenig and Cohen (2002: 115).

Among some subsets of the American population, religious participation has been found to be a stronger determinant of psychological well-being than either health or wealth. The most robust data pertains to life satisfaction among African Americans, particularly black elders. The recent suicide rate among black men over 65 is one-third that of their white peers. Nearly 5 out of every 100,000 older white women took their lives in 1998; only 20 black women over 65 committed suicide in the entire country that year (Conwell, 2002). Religiosity buffers the consequences of negative events by increasing actual and subjective sources of social support, by enhancing persons' self-esteem and sense of control, by reducing the risks of marital discord and legal problems, by enabling individuals to increase their capacity for problem solving, and by regulating their emotions (Ellison, 1998; Levin, 2001: 3).

The relationship between religion and disability has also been analyzed. Among people with disabilities, more than two-thirds prayed for their own health, compared to the half surveyed who were not impaired. Women more often than men pray for their own healthfulness, though the percentage of both sexes who do so increases with age. Women with disabilities, moreover, are more likely than disabled men to seek pastoral care. Both sexes at all ages are more inclined to take this step than those without disabilities (Hendershot, 2002a, b). Prayer and the benefit of clergy may give strength in infirmity, but it does not always result in recovery. John Paul II, aged 83, had to be wheeled to the ceremony celebrating the twenty-fifth year of his papacy. A victim of Parkinson's disease, his left hand trembled uncontrollably, and his head drooped. The head of Christendom's largest church intended to give hope to others by not hiding his mortality (Bruni, 2003).

There is a growing literature on how faith-based psychosocial and behavioral interventions impact various acute diseases, such as breast cancer and malignant melanoma. While acknowledging that more information needs to be gathered, scientists have reported cases in which religion (and the hope and social support that go with it) has helped victims of such autoimmune diseases as AIDS, rheumatoid arthritis, psoriasis, diabetes, lupus erythematosus, and chronic fatigue syndrome, all maladies in which an overactive immune system attacks otherwise healthy tissue (Koenig and Cohen, 2002: 6–7).

Jeffrey Levin, who as a graduate student established a field he called the "epidemiology of religion," uncovered case studies buried in the medical literature that anticipated current research. Levin (1994: 4–7) collected 250 studies published over a 150-year period that met rigorous contemporary tests of reliability. To this he added geriatric and gerontological articles and survey data that touched on the mental and physical consequences of religious involvement. Levin's collection showed that religion made a difference in the treatment and outcome of dozens of other diseases, ranging from myocardial infarction, hypertension, and emphysema, to tuberculosis (Levin, 2001: 31). On the basis of his research, Levin postulates that religious affiliation benefits health by

- promoting healthy behavior and lifestyles
- buffering the effects of stress and isolation
- strengthening the physiological effects of positive emotions
- reinforcing health-promoting personality styles
- nurturing hope, optimism, and positive expectations
- activating an altered state of consciousness
- invoking paranormal means of healing others. (2001: 13–14)

Many investigators suspect that Levin is way ahead of the curve in presenting his last two postulates, but the meticulous quality of his epidemiological investigations legitimizes the field, encouraging others to follow his lead.

To the extent that faith-based beliefs and activities complement the principles of preventive medicine, healthful lifestyles, and personalities that can cope with the vicissitudes of daily living, researchers have amassed evidence intimating that religiosity may prolong life. Follow-up studies of those who attend services regularly seem to indicate a longevity advantage over nonobservers, after taking age, health, functioning, social support, and psychological profile into account (*American Journal of Public Health*, 1998; Duke University, 1999). That 90 percent of older U.S. adults put great stock in the power of religion underscores its centrality to consumers' sense of well-being (Koenig and Cohen, 2002: 12). The association among religious involvement, healthfulness, and lower mortality rates appears stronger among women than men (Strawbridge et al., 1997). No reputable researcher yet has declared definitively that religious beliefs and practices extend healthful longevity. Critics note that most studies fail to control for obesity, which is now recognized to be a leading cause of death after the age of 50. And scientists trained in orthodox methods plead for studying the mechanisms through which religious engagement seems positively correlated with mortality rates (McCullough et al., 2000: 14, 16).

Institutions of higher learning are developing research agenda and teaching classes to buttress efforts made by faith-based organizations to build on associations between religion and healthful aging. At the University of Minnesota, older students interested in complementary medicine and holistic health care can take classes sponsored since 1995 through the university's ElderLearning Institute and the Center for Spirituality and Healing (Center for Spirituality and Healing, 2004). Paralleling the efforts of the National Organization for Empowering Caregivers, Ohio State University's College of Family and Consumer Sciences proposes faith-based, familial rituals that make transitions to retirement or a nursing home less stressful (Shriner, 1996; see also Cibuzar, n.d.; G. Mitchell, 1999).

Virtually every tradition justifies giving high priority to using ancient and novel texts and practices to enhance vital aging, especially in later years. Jewish renewal, according to Michael Lerner, presupposes that "no communal transformation is real unless it involves individual healing and repair, and no individual healing can be sustained unless it is associated with communal transformation" (1994: 357). The New Testament abounds in stories of the healing power of faith: Jesus and his apostles cured people who were blind, deaf, mute, lame, or near death. One's status increases with age in Muslim society, in part because the Koran insists that followers honor and respect the old, supporting them in infirmity as much as possible. Confucianism also puts great stress on filial piety; neglecting one's elders, in turn, brings shame (Ritts, 2000: 16, 18). Buddhism teaches that suffering is inevitable. Still, like other major religions, Buddhism asks children to support their parents in old age, and it expects elderly people to provide a suitable inheritance (Della Santina, 1987: 4–5). For tradition's sake and for purposes of renewal, faith-based communities should do four things:

First, they should *expand the usage of religious texts and practices that sustain physical and mental well-being* (Achenbaum, 1995a). Faith communities might encourage congregants to read the sacred literature of other religious congregations. "Like desire," observes bell hooks (1994: 167), "language disrupts, refuses to be contained within boundaries." Reading passages that are not part of the repertoire freshens the power of familiar words to comfort and heal. Some people seek more radical alternatives to supplement what their congregations offer. All sorts of claims are made for the healing powers of foot reflexology, crystal therapy, charkas, meridians, LightBody, Reiki, herbal therapies, and dreamtime interpretations (Awakening-Healing, 2004; Star-Gates, 2004). Few medical researchers or clergy endorse these latter forms of "divine tune-up." They may not cause harm, nor are they proved to relieve suffering. It is better for older persons to rely on religious practices that complement their traditional observances.

Hence, second, faith communities should *stress the value of prayer, for oneself and for others, in late life*. Prayer may resemble what Levin characterizes as a "paranormal phenomena," but it is more than that (Apologetics Index, 2001). Most congregations recite, during their weekly services, the names of individuals within the congregation or known by congregants to be sick or in need and solicit prayers in their behalf. It is equally important that prayers be offered in thanksgiving. As Adi Granth, a Sikh, put it: "Of all the prayers of the heart, the best prayer is the prayer to the Master to be given the grace of properly praising the Lord" (International Religious Foundation, 1995: 594). Having experienced most of the joys and tribulations that can occur over the life course, elderly persons are in a privileged position. They can meditate daily in gratitude for the fruits of creation, good and bad.

Third, *healing services should become a more regular and more visible religious ritual*. In the Episcopal Church, for instance, time is apportioned during certain Eucharistic services for participants to come forward, ask a priest for intercessions, and then receive an anointing and a blessing. Lay ministers or clergy visit the homebound, bearing consolatory words, communion, and oils. Not surprisingly, people middle-aged and older are more likely to participate in healing services than are younger individuals. Healing services provide a way to include older congregants in the life of the faith community, thereby restoring the health of the participant and the institution alike. Feminist liturgies should be designed for services frequented by older women (Procter-Smith, 1995).

Ideally, parishes have a senior ministry, but few attend to older people as assiduously as they do to families with young children whom they wish to recruit and retain in the fold. Healing services can provide an outward sign of the congregation's concern for its older members.

Finally, religious communities should *pay more attention to the spiritual health of its membership, especially older ones.* William James wrote in *The Varieties of Religious Experience* about "subconsciously maturing processes eventuating in results of which we suddenly grow conscious" (1902: 203). "The potentialities of development in human souls are unfathomable," he said (349). Spiritual development is not identical to religious maturity, but the two spheres are complementary. Engagement in a religious context often facilitates spiritual growth (Hitchcock, 1991: 28). In recent decades, baby boomers have been paying more attention to the inward depths and outward manifestations of their spiritual development. Their coming of age religiously, argues Jeff Levin, "coincided with the social upheaval of the 1960s, the human potential movement of the 1970s, and the growth of Eastern and New Age beliefs in the 1980s. . . . Daily meditation or incorporation of contemplative elements into traditional rituals, more so than weekly church or synagogue attendance, is the most typical expression of this spiritual path" (2001: 155). Levin sees the analysis of spiritual practices as the next frontier for the epidemiology of religion.

At the individual level, the varieties of spiritual experiences attest to the manifold ways in which men and women encounter the immanent and transcendent dimensions of their relationship with the Divine. Collectively, spiritual elders derive from their inner depths gifts of discernment that often move them to take bold social, political, and economic action in the secular realm (Leech, 1992). Religious organizations thus should cultivate the spiritual lives of their aging members as a vital component of their healthful longevity. Ripeness disciplines them "to do justice, and to love kindness, and to walk humbly with [their] God" (Micah 6:8).

The Varieties of Spiritual Insights and Experiences

Invitations to spiritual awakening are recorded in the foundational texts of all faith traditions. Chuang Tzu, a Chinese Taoist who lived in the fourth century B.C.E., wrote poems full of spiritual imagery that became a source of inspiration for Thomas Merton, one of the most influential Christian spiritual leaders of the twentieth century (Palmer, 1999: 36–38). Spirituality undergirds Christianity. Jesus went into the wilderness to pray and fast before he began his ministry (Matthew 4:1–11). His followers manifested spiritual fruits in diverse ways in the early years of the Jesus movement (Acts 1:8, 9:17, 11:16). "Spiritual gifts," noted St. Paul, range from wisdom, knowledge, healing, working miracles, prophecy, and discernment, to interpretation of languages (1 Corinthians 12:1–11; Ephesians 4:11–12). Different people possess different gifts, but they all ultimately contribute to serving the Lord in love (1 Corinthians 13).

Nor is the Western appropriation of Eastern spirituality a recent phenomenon. Apollonus went to India in 220 C.E. to learn from "wise men marked with a crescent on their foreheads" (Irwin, 2004: 13). Swedenborgians in the 1840s combined interests in Mesmerism, Eastern notions of reincarnation, and ideas indigenous to their founders; by 1850 they had formed 150 Spiritualist circles in New York alone. Twenty-five years later, William Judge, Henry Steel Olcott, and Russian psychic Helena Petrovna Blavatsky formed the Theosophical Society as a "universal brotherhood" to explore how Eastern and Western religions, ancient and modern, nurtured latent psychic powers in human beings (ibid.: 23, 25).

Spiritual quests, while often emanating out of formal religious practices, nonetheless have a life of their own. They manage to meld seemingly alien traditions into highly personal visions. No wonder contemporary spirituality in the United States is so compatible with the eclectic, pluralist dynamics of American religiosity. Both seek fresh styles of thought, feeling, and behavior that embody people's innermost being. They resonate with postmodern sensibilities, conjoining an appreciation for the theological relativity of icons with a willingness to engage by turns in "festive" play and in solitary contemplation. In kindling the spark of the Divine within, spiritual exercises eschew solipsism; instead, they simultaneously invite pilgrims to embrace the interrelatedness of humans with all that is ennobling and horrific on earth and beyond. Spirituality engenders compassion, "a quality that makes action responsive rather than reflexive" (Palmer, 1999: 123; see also Cox, 1968).

Current cohorts of older Americans have become intrigued by the spiritual dimensions of their existence. As they review their accomplishments and failures, and as they face their own finitude, elderly people seek ways to affix meaning to past experiences, present circumstances, and future prospects. Some write memoirs or assemble photographs. Others create memory gardens or give away mementos (*Generations*, 1998). Through the creation and distribution of these legacies, many older people seek a means of spiritual assistance that allays their doubts and fears as it helps them appreciate what they have accomplished over the years. In affirming their faith in God and humankind, they search for ways to attain peace and knowledge and to map pathways toward closure. There is ample precedent for this contemporary phenomenon: Ignatius of Loyola, after all, designed his *Spiritual Exercises* for persons who had to make life-and-death decisions (Jewell, 1999: 15, 29). Older women are particularly imaginative in crafting spiritual practices that combine meditation with art, that involve them in soul-searching through gender-based rituals, and that nourish friendships.

Recently, Americans have created institutions to capture the essence of late-life spirituality. This typically has been the nation's way of grounding even esoteric concepts since the early decades of the Republic. Alexis de Tocqueville stressed the importance of voluntary associations in *Democracy in America*:

> In no country in the world has the principle of association been more successfully used or applied to a greater multitude of objects than in America. Besides the permanent associations which are established by law under the names of townships, cities, and countries, a vast number of others are formed and maintained by the agency of private individuals. . . . In the United States associations are established to promote the public safety, commerce, industry, morality, and religion. There is no end which the human will despairs of attaining through the combined power of individuals united into a society. . . . An association consists simply in the public assent which a number of individuals give to certain doctrines and in the engagement which they contract to promote in a certain manner the spread of those doctrines. (1836c: 1:198–99)

Spirituality by definition has no doctrinal basis: individuals choose what works best for them among a plethora of ideas and practices. But even in the pursuit of intimate spiritual matters, Americans are inclined to join and drop out of associations with which they alternately feel affinity or disaffection.

Public assent to institutionalize late-life spirituality was evident among delegates to the first White House Conference on Aging (1961), who made nearly a thousand recommendations addressing the spiritual concerns of older Americans. At the second White House Conference on Aging in 1971, delegates formed a National Interfaith Coalition on Aging (NICA), to serve as an umbrella organization for more than one hundred Protestant, Catholic, Jewish, and nondenominational bodies. In 1991, NICA became a constituent unit of the National Council on the Aging. The American Society on Aging created a counterpart, a Forum on Religion and Aging (1988), to share models of faith-based practices and spiritual models with its membership (Kimble et al., 1995: 212).

Religious leaders have established independent centers for men and women seeking to deepen the spiritual dimensions of their lives. In 1984 Rabbi Zalman Schacter-Shalomi, then in his mid-60s, took a forty-day "vision-quest retreat" to overcome his depression over lost youth, unresolved problems, and anxiety over what the future held. Like many of his older contemporaries, Schacter-Shalomi felt that he was "living in the box of the unlived life." The rabbi returned home both refreshed and convinced that he had to help to transform negative attitudes toward old age and aging. "Having come to face our mortality, having been reconciled, we still can close our eyes and, in our imagination, look at the fuel gauge of available time. Most of us find that we still have some mileage left" (Schacter-Shalomi, 2004).

Based on ideas about the roles of tribal elders, influenced by developments in "brain-mind" research, and impressed by the fervor and tactics of environmentalists, Rabbi Schacter-Shalomi established a nonprofit, multifaith educational site called the Spiritual Eldering Institute in Boulder, Colorado, in 1989. Initial support came from private donors, gerontologists, and ALEPH (the Alliance for Jewish Renewal). When his book, *From Ageing to Sage-ing* (1995) became a bestseller, the public took closer note of Schacter-Shalomi's blueprint for spiritual growth in later years. The Spiritual Eldering Institute is "dedicated to the spiritual dimensions of aging and conscious living, to affirming the importance of the elder years, and to teaching individuals how to harvest their life's wisdom and transform it into a legacy for future generations." A major priority is training leaders and professionals to extend the Institute's mission to other parts of the country. The rabbi wants partnerships with groups committed to promoting growth through "conscious aging." More than one hundred "Sage-ing leaders" have been trained; "Sage-ing" centers have been established in South Bend, Indiana, and several sites in Florida (Spiritual Eldering Institute, 2004; Enfield and Formichelli, 2005).

Schacter-Shalomi's references to tribal elders remind us that aged people of various ethnic and racial groups have been mobilized institutionally to serve as role models for members of their own communities and society at large. Native Americans, who ascribe to spiritual wisdom in late life, have networks beyond their reservations. Bookstore chains distribute publications imparting the insights of wise tribal men and women. Representatives from twenty-one tribes in North and Central America formed the Spiritual Elders of Mother Earth in 2000 to create a legacy for the next seven generations: "Our children's generations that are coming are waiting for this gift. . . . So we are going to have to hold hands and go in one direction. All of us have to communicate, sing one song, say one prayer, and walk the next decade with one voice, for survival and the survival of future generations" (Spiritual Elders of Mother Earth, 2004). The diverse voices of Cherokees, Mayans, Oglala Sioux, and Coahuilteco/Huicho, among others, spiritually unite in a common prayer and united purpose.

Spirituality reinforces black consciousness among African Americans. "By creating a context for the creation and expression of black soul culture, African-American spirituality has engendered a model of human freedom that differs from all others" (Stewart, 1999: 1). Older African Americans play a central role in telling their stories as well as those of their natural and fictive kin. Elders guide the faithful in all aspects of life. The special status accorded to the wisdom of age in the black community is longstanding. African-American spirituality remembers the brutality of slavery and oppression in the United States and in Africa in order to acknowledge how divine power imparts resilience in the face of prejudice and inhumanity. Songs and prayers empower participants with a will to survive, and more than that, to create spiritual idioms that inspire them to thrive. It is not by accident that spirituals such as "Were You There When They Crucified My Lord" are sung in cathedrals and white Protestant parishes as well as in store-front black congregations during Holy Week. The lugubrious strains, born out of human suffering yet mindful of God's redemptive power, harmonize disparate historical events and cultural backdrops into a powerful set of widely held emotions.

In the domain of "trans-traditional spirituality" (Bianchi, 1997) are to be found expressions of creative elderhood predisposed to spiritual wisdom wherever it presents itself. Life reviews written at advanced ages affirm the human potential to select and integrate meanings and metaphors from sources as disparate in time and space as religious folk art, popular music, Taoist meditations, and theoretical physics. Traversing the gulf that frequently exists between the secular and the sacred in contemporary society, spiritual journeys become ways of reweaving frayed strands of individual life histories, of connecting one's inward being with the experiences of others (including strangers), and of relating to nature in all its compositions.

Not surprisingly, intergenerational organizations have sprung up to facilitate the process. The RUAH Spirituality Institute, launched in Brookline, Massachusetts, in 2002, promotes interfaith dialogue addressing spirituality and aging, healing, spirituality and the environment, grief and dying, and mysticism. "RUAH aims to increase understanding among religious traditions, provide spiritual sustenance to all, and to create peace one person at a time" (RUAH, 2004). "One Light, Many Lamps" is the motto of the SHEM Center for Interfaith Spirituality in Oak Park, Illinois. Its program, which extends a welcome to gays, lesbians, and those questioning their sexual orientation, includes chants, dancing, and retreats as well as canoe trips and camping, "where words are born of silence, a place where the whispers of the heart arise" (SHEM, 2004).

Many trans-spiritual groups that have taken shape in the United States are gender specific. According to a poll by AARP, nearly half of all women surveyed—compared to about a third of male respondents—said that they sought spiritual growth (Business Women's Network, 2002: 153). Spiritual discussions occur over a kitchen table and transpire as women quilt or prepare for a ballet class. Others take place through the auspices of faith-based organizations. Various congregations offer yoga sessions, prayer services, Bible study, classes in Eastern and Western mysticism, and volunteer activities, which are especially valued by retirees. Retreats are popular because they afford opportunities for women to have quiet time to themselves, punctuated with moments to share with one another how their spirituality gives meaning to their lives.

A Roman Catholic Bishop's Committee on Women in Society and in the Church (2003), focusing on persons over 40, reported that spirituality helped women integrate their work and family responsibilities in creative ways. Resisting the male tendency to compartmentalize roles, many women declared that they lived out their spiritual beliefs in the workplace. Some pointedly noted that their bosses appreciated and used their gifts and skills more than the church did (U.S. Conference of Catholic Bishops, 2003a: 2–5).

Men's spiritual groups serve to foster fellowship, to strengthen spirituality through prayer and sacraments, and to do good works. In some ways, men's spiritual centers face greater obstacles than those for women, because many males are not as comfortable as females with disclosing their fears and hopes to one another. Self-discovery, while important for personal growth, does not motivate all individuals to engage with a community of peers willing to listen to their stories and affirm their value. Thus, many congregations offer communal options to older men. The Roman Catholic Church has established a national network of ministries, a clearinghouse for information, and training programs under the auspices of the National Resource Center for Catholic Men (Hauprich, 2004; U.S. Conference of Catholic Bishops, 2003b). Some secular groups, like the New Warriors, borrow heavily from Native American traditions and Jungian psychology to help members come to terms with their successes and failures and to prepare them to serve "ManKind."

Common to these initiatives supporting male spirituality is the premise that concepts of masculinity are undergoing change. Faith-based communities and secular organizations recognize that it is important for older men who have wrestled with issues of identity, power, and morality to mentor boys and youth so that they may in due course become spiritually mature men. Intergenerational lessons, imparted through rites of passage, include messages such as "Life is hard," "You are going to die," and "Your life is not about you" (Rohr, 1998; Levine, 2001).

Promise Keepers is probably the best known (and most controversial) men's group; it aims to "promote spiritual revival in the homes, churches, and communities of this nation." Founded in 1990, the organization stages stadium rallies, offers seminars, and sells books and videos to motivate men "toward Christ-like masculinity" (Promise Keepers, 1999). That it attracted 725,000 men to rallies in 1995 alone attests to the success of Promise Keepers in satisfying the spiritual yearning of men from diverse backgrounds (Center for Democracy Studies, 1996: 1). Elderly men are essential to the network because all participants must have an older mentor with whom to bond and to be accountable. The influence of this so-called "folk religion" has been waning since the late 1990s, in part because of internal politics, in part because of charges of sexism in its message. The National Organization for Women, among other groups, criticizes Promise Keepers as a radically right-wing organization that is homophobic and too insistent in spreading St. Paul's dictum that "wives be subject to their husbands" (Titus 2: 3–5; National Organization for Women, 2004).

The spiritually hungry also turn to standard and alternative forms of therapy to help them (re)construct their identities. Forty percent of all Americans participate in a small-group setting that meets regularly to provide care and support (Steere, 1997: 27; Spickard, 1995). "Stay connected with people on your own wavelength," recommends gerontologist H. R. Moody, to get the support to develop an inner self (quoted in Cutter, 2003: 3). Members of professional organizations such as the American Psychological Association (APA) and the American Counseling Association (ACA) agree about the importance of introducing a spiritual dimension into counseling. The APA's Division 36, the Psychology of Religion, had roughly 1,200 members in 2000; the ACA's Association for Spiritual, Ethical, and Religious Values in Counseling had 2,700 members. The latter organization has added spirituality to its accreditation guidelines. Other groups, such as the Academy of Religion and Mental Health (1954), have merged professional interests instead of creating special interest groups (G. Miller, 2003: 3, 33).

Although spirituality is not as extensively analyzed as the associations between religion and healthful aging, some healthcare professionals and their patients see reason to introduce it into mainstream medicine. Some wellness programs for older adults emphasize the spiritual dimensions of fitness, inviting elders to ponder life's big questions as they exercise and dance. Yoga has become the number one activity among consumers; more than half of all fitness centers offered yoga classes in 2002 (Milner, 2002: 58; see also Bleakney, 1994 and Jurek, 1996). Early research suggests a connection between the brain and spirituality; brain tumors, which overexcite the limbic system, spark spiritual awareness in some patients (Orloff, 2001). Expanding previous studies that identified the contribution spirituality made to psychological well being in older adults, a team of British scholars recently demonstrated that spirituality also moderated some of the negative effects of frailty (Kirby et al., 2004: P123–29). Increased spiritual well-being has also been correlated with lower anxiety about death, particularly among cancer victims (National Cancer Institute, 2004; RVY, 2000).

Without question, of all the health-based spiritual initiatives, Alcoholics Anonymous (AA) has had the greatest impact in the United States. Its roots can be traced back to Benjamin Rush, who recognized alcoholism as a disease that needed to be treated; to the writings of Carl Jung and William James; and to the Oxford Movement, a group of Protestant pietistic evangelicals who in the early twentieth century believed that public confession and spiritual conversion enabled people to overcome addiction (Kurtz, 1979: 33–34, 180–82). Founded by Bill Wilson and Dr. Bob Smith, AA had reached 133,000 men and women who had read its publications and attended its meetings within twenty years. Alcoholics Anonymous claims that its 12-step program—which stresses the need for self-examination, personal responsibility, reliance on God, apologies to those harmed by the wrong-doing, and, finally, "a spiritual awakening as a result of these steps"—has helped more than two million problem drinkers to recover (Primedia, 2004; Alcoholics Anonymous, 2004). AA's model has been adapted by other organizations interested in helping individuals recover from various addictions.

Because of its diverse roots and tenacious adherence to a prescribed set of rules for meetings and for individuals' code of behavior, the ways that Alcoholics Anonymous is characterized depend on situational contexts. The organization's invocation of a Higher Power is made as generic as possible to reach all people in need. Thus, a nun who regularly attends AA meetings debunks notions that AA depends on New Age mysticism or panders to self-indulgence: in *Seeds of Grace,* "Sister Molly" draws connections to Catholic meditation and prayer (Haller, 1998; Park Ridge Center, 2001). And while many Mexican Americans find themselves both culturally alienated from the United States and marginalized by their kin because of their excessive drinking, they feel comfortable participating in Alcoholics Anonymous. There are 720 Spanish-speaking groups listed in the AA General Service Board. People attend AA meetings regardless of class or ethnicity; there are now more chapters outside the United States than within (K. Davis, 1994: 8, 23, 95).

Alcohol abuse is most prevalent between the ages of 18 and 44 and far more common among men than women. Treatment programs as well as social and health factors reduce the prevalence of alcoholism, especially among those over 75. Still, because alcoholism is a progressive (often undetected) disease, it is not surprising that a tenth of all adult alcoholics in the United States are over 60. Since it is never too late to strive for long-term abstinence, many older Americans turn to AA with the support of their families (Manheimer, 1994: 463–64; Schick and Schick, 1994: 103). Authentic spirituality demands action, not only in overcoming addiction but also in confronting other personal and societal problems.

Spirituality Spurs Social Action in Later Years

Spirituality, unlike philosophy or theology, requires that meditations result in actions, deeds that enliven intimate engagements in the world. "True contemplation is never a mere retreat," claims Parker Palmer in *The Active Life*. "Instead, it draws us deeper into right action by getting us more deeply in touch with the gifts that we have to give, with our need to give them, with the people and problems that need us" (1999: 122). Spiritual awakenings summon us to be "citizen pilgrims," working to make the world better. They prepare us to challenge and criticize the destructive tendencies of our individual and collective activities (Griffin, 1988: 91; Solomon, 2002; Miller and Cook-Greuter, 2000).

Spiritual elders are ideally positioned to play the role of citizen pilgrims in creative ways. Having lived through tumultuous political, social, economic, and moral changes in their local communities and in other parts of the world, they can apply the lessons of the past in charting the general direction of future developments. Like everybody else, aged people are caught in a web of forces only partially in their control. This is why resiliency and adaptability are critical with advancing years. Previous chapters have documented the ability of countless older men and women to re-create meaningful identities after their full-time careers end, to utilize educational practices and opportunities that exist outside formal institutions of higher learning, and to adapt healthful habits in the face of the indifference of healthcare professionals. In the opinion of ecologist Thomas Berry, America's old people understand the choice before them: "They participate either as positive contributors or as negative burdens to the community and to the earth. While their mode of participation may be changed, their presence and their insights, their energy, their influence are demanded" (2001: 3). The wisdom of age required today need not be packaged in an elegant treatise or heroic efforts. For the sake of the human community, we seek the sustained creativity of ordinary men and women who put a premium on vouchsafing the fundamentals of the human condition because they are all too aware that time is short.

Aging religious figures such as Rabbi Schacter-Shalomi serve as role models. There are others. Rabbi Leonard Beerman, semi-retired from the most prominent temple in Los Angeles, remains highly visible on boards committed to social justice. Co-founder of the Interfaith Center to Reverse the Arms Race, co-chair of the Los Angeles Jewish Commission on Sweatshops, Beerman also serves on the Blue Ribbon Committee for Affordable Housing in Los Angeles. "Jewish optimism is rooted in the profound contempt for life as it is. If you don't have that contempt for life as it is, you are not an optimist. Because you can imagine the way of life different from the one you live in, that's optimism" (Stanczak and Miller, 2002: 5). Joan Chittister, the former prioress of the Benedictine Sisters of Erie, Pennsylvania, and author of several standard works on Benedictine spirituality, founded Benetvision to find "bridges between private and public spirituality . . . Benetvision is designed to look at both of those levels of the person in the relationship to the religious impulse" (ibid.: 54). Acting on her spiritual insights, Chittister plays an active role in the International Peace Council. Under its auspices, she has traveled to more than three dozen countries on behalf of human rights issues. The Rev. William A. Lawson served forty-two years as founding pastor of Wheeler Baptist Church in Houston, Texas. Under his leadership, it grew from 13 men and women meeting in a living room to a complex serving more than 4,500 members, with services held in three buildings via closed-circuit TV. Lawson worked closely with Dr. Martin Luther King Jr. during the latter's last three years of life, became deeply involved in community development, and established a middle school to help African-American youth develop character. Now, at 78, Lawson is overseeing a fifty-unit housing project for senior citizens (Vara, 2004). Finally, Dr. Mansur Khan represents a new generation of leaders of Islamic centers and mosques who deplored the unwillingness of fellow congregants to go out of the community. Besides generously contributing funds to Muslims in Third World countries, he also offers his healthcare skills to poor people in his neighborhood (Stanczak and Miller, 2002: 5).

These four exemplars have three things in common. First, their spirituality is intentional, translating private meditations into a diverse mix of public concerns. Second, they act: they engage in civic affairs to bring about change. Third, they are open to working through organizational structures of their own making or ones that already exist (ibid.: 53).

Spiritually and religiously inclined elders do not have to be movers and shakers to make a difference. They do not need to aspire to national prominence. They can begin in their own family circle and in their neighborhoods by bridging the gap that presently exists in too many instances between the activities of organized religion and the private realm of spirituality. "Coming out of one's cocoon in the public sphere is just as necessary to self-realization as it is in the private," argues Paul Rogat Loeb in *Soul of a Citizen* (1999: 22). Once ordinary elders take the first step and reach out, they will undoubtedly find themselves in the midst of others, transforming educational institutions, healthcare networks, and the marketplaces of producers and consumers. Naturally, men and women who do not wish to spend their remaining years as "givers" have the right to pursue other activities. But it is incumbent on them at least to articulate a vision of the "good society" (and its deficiencies) for those who want to listen to what they have to say. Through telling their life stories, through sharing the fruits of their lives, older men and women can instill a set of values into the public square ripe enough for rising generations to harvest.

Extending the Civic Engagement of Senior Citizens } 6

According to the *Oxford English Dictionary,* the noun *senior* has been used since the twelfth century to refer to "an elder person . . . superior or worthy of deference and reverence by reason of age." The term *senior citizen,* in contrast, first appeared in the October 24, 1938, issue of *Time* magazine: "Mr. Downey had an inspiration to do something on behalf of what he calls, for campaign purposes, 'our senior citizens.'"

Both the *Oxford English Dictionary* and *The American Heritage Book of English Usage* attribute other ascriptions to "senior citizen." The *OED* notes that the British employ the term in "official communications" to refer to pensioners. In American English, a "senior citizen" has attained "retirement" age though is not necessarily retired. *American Heritage* adds that "*senior citizen* denotes not only age but also social or civic status, making it the natural term to use when discussing an older person in a political or social context."

"Senior citizen" gained currency as increasing numbers of elders and associations representing their interests grew more active in the public arena (Flexner, 1982: 478; K. Wilson, 1993). "Senior" attested to a person's years of experience, whereas "senior citizens" referred to the younger segment of the 50+ population, especially those who provided direct services to their communities or received them through agencies. "It's the first term to acknowledge the old as a political constituency" (Nunberg, 2004: 7; see also Kokkola, 1998: 2; National Academy for

Teaching and Learning about Aging, 1999; Gergen and Gergen, 2004; Yadurajan, 2004). Thus, "senior citizen" would seem to be the ideal term to use in this chapter treating the political dimensions of population aging.

Alas, the etymology is not as straightforward as the preceding commentary suggests. Barely half of all men and women of a certain age, reports Betty Friedan, use "senior citizen" to describe themselves (1993: 36; see also Berman, 1981). Baby boomers find the term biased and unflattering (Bestler, 2004; Kaiser, 2004). Still, it is preferable to other options. Only 8 percent of those over 65 consider "old" an acceptable designation, according to the *American Heritage Dictionary*. A majority of elders also object to "older Americans," "old-timers," and "aged persons," which in their opinion convey a sense of frailty and dependency. And calling someone "retired" insinuates economic uselessness (Kokkola, 1998).

Both "seniors" and "senior citizens," in short, have "unpleasantly euphemistic" connotations (*AskOxford,* 2004: 4). Editorial stylists recommend that the labels be used "carefully and sparingly," not as a substitute for "elderly" (Garbl's Writing Center, 2004; see also *Plain Language,* 2004: 19). The term *senior citizen* was omitted as an entry from the three leading lexicons prepared by gerontologists. Nor does it appear in the first two editions of the *Encyclopedia of Aging* (National Institutes of Health, 1986; Harris, 1988; Maddox, 1995; Achenbaum, Weiland, and Haber, 1996: 124, 128). "The shelf life of a euphemism is short. . . . Pretty soon, the stigma catches up with the label, infects it, and then the euphemism breaks down" (Wajnryb, 2003).

No alternative to "senior citizens" has yet arisen to define older political actors. "Golden agers" is a popular though apolitical euphemism (*OED online*). "Seasoned citizens" has been proposed (Kaiser, 2004) to describe the "suddenly senior," but the term has not yet entered common parlance or dictionaries. "Veteranship," argues Douglas Nelson, conveys a sense of respect for old age, comparable to that accorded youth and middle age. "Veteranship" affords older people support that empowers their right to self-determination, enhances their authority or prestige in conducting their lives, and in the policy arena values their input concerning their needs and capabilities. Yet Nelson questions "whether 'veteranship' contains enough concrete political and social meaning to offer a practical point of view for aging policy" (1982: 163).

Absent a better choice, this chapter, which surveys the civic engagement of older people, uses the term *senior citizens* to underscore the rights and responsibilities of men and women in advancing age. Special attention is paid to a citizen's call to service in the latter portion of the life course (Dowell, 1998; Wajnryb, 2003). "An active, effective and responsible citizenship, in contemporary times, requires that people be empowered to exercise those rights and responsibilities towards other people, the community, and the state," declared Ana Maria Ramalho Correia in a white paper for UNESCO. "Citizens should be vigilant regarding the responsiveness of the state towards them and the members of their community and should be motivated to participate in public life" (2002: 1).

Population aging invites senior citizens to assume heretofore under-valued and underused roles as a political constituency for the sake of societal well-being. They have a responsibility to impart their wisdom to rising generations. A lifetime of experiences should spark a passion for humanitarian causes, which in turn obliges old people at times to engage in direct political action. Conversely, as Paul Rogat Loeb notes, "When we shrink from the world, our souls shrink too" (1999: 23). Senior citizens in decades ahead must become advocates of global priorities; political actors at the national, state, and local levels as well as kin resources; and individual role models of civility. Not all senior citizens will aspire to positions of leadership. Many prefer interacting with family and friends to promoting international causes. In the short term, senior citizens' initial civic involvement will probably be localized, where their contributions are vitally necessary (Center for Third Age Leadership, 2004). With time, their horizons ideally will broaden.

Politically effective senior citizens are discerning in their commitments. Many have learned to distinguish between what they have come to know matters and what does not. Followers are as essential as leaders in assessing and transforming global, national, communal, and familial bonds. Political engagement at any level requires courage—courage to assume responsibility, courage to serve, courage to challenge, courage to participate in transformation, courage to take moral action, and courage to insist that leaders listen to their constituencies (Wills, 1994; Chaleff, 2003: 6–7). Above all, the politics of senior citizenship requires confidence and hope—confidence that younger persons will join their initiatives, and hope that some good will result from engaging in this relatively unexplored arena.

In his book *Senescence,* 78-year-old G. Stanley Hall affirmed the potential of elders as political actors even before the term "senior citizen" was coined:

> Perhaps in the large Aristotelian sense of the word, politics is, par excellence, the work of and for old age. . . . If the young are the best advocates, the old are by nature the best judges. They can best weigh facts and ideas in the scales of justice. The moral faculties ripen more slowly. Thus the old can best supplement the technicalities of law by equity and give ethics its rights in their verdicts. They should be the keepers of the standards of right and wrong and mete out justice with the impartiality and aloofness that befit it. Even in private life we have a judicial function, which, though often ignored and resented, is also sought and respected if we have the tact to praise and do not become censorious. . . . [T]he supreme criterion of everything, including religion, science, art, property, business, education, hygiene, and every human institution and everything in our environment, is what it contributes to make life longer, fuller, and saner, so that each individual will live out more completely all the essentials in the life of the race. (1922: 424–26)

Hall's prescient plea for greater civic engagement by senior citizens to complement the work of younger and middle-aged people has special meaning today. More than ever, we must rely on the ripeness of age to actualize genuinely disinterested public service.

Global Aging

Americans throughout much of their national experience, believing themselves insulated by geography and good fortune from the machinations that caused turmoil elsewhere, have tended either to look inward or to impose their worldview on the international scene. Those over 50 should know that neither option works. Learning from the past, they can attest to the interdependency of nations. Senior citizens can illuminate how international environmental, political, and humanitarian problems shape domestic circumstances.

In the colonial era and early years of the Republic, we were an outpost, largely ignored by European potentates. Yet even then immigration, slavery, trade, and fights of territorial expansion insinuated the United States into global affairs. Isolationists, internationalists, jingoists, moralists, and pragmatists a century later competed to articulate U.S. foreign policy (Martin et al., 2000). Matters at home typically took priority; Americans focused on crises abroad if and when they threatened domestic tranquility.

Our parents, whom journalists characterize as "the Great Generation," were the first cohort to experience the never-ending travails and full horrors of this country's engagement on the world arena. Amid a worldwide depression, U.S. leaders initially made little effort to stop the aggression and violation of human rights in Europe and Asia. After World War II, the Great Generation tried to apply the global lessons they had learned, while concentrating on their children, their jobs, and their friends.

The United States designed a cold war strategy that did not always fit the real challenges of the day (Neustadt and May, 1986). Convinced that communists resembled fascists, Americans by and large responded to the postcolonial brutalities as if they were facets of the Manichean struggle between two major powers. The United States underestimated nations' capacity (including its own) to defy basic standards of decent conduct. American Jews at first denied the significance of the Holocaust (Novick, 1999). Christians rarely referred to the atrocity; they could not apprehend how civilized peoples could perpetrate such evil. Similarly, Americans justified the devastation of Hiroshima and Nagasaki because atom bombs ended the war in the Pacific sooner than traditional means would have (Dower, 1999). The stage was set for others to develop equally lethal deterrents.

To keep peace and to prosper internationally, the Great Generation relied in part on the United Nations to intervene when bloodshed, revolutions, hatred, ignorance, and prejudice threatened our world order. Americans contributed to organizations such as the International Red Cross to engage in relief efforts abroad. The Great Generation believed that such political and humanitarian institutions as well as its military prowess could contain communist forces while promoting democratic self-determination in new nations. Intellectuals and political commentators during the 1950s and 1960s celebrated the fruits of American exceptionalism. Others sought to rectify "an American dilemma" that denied blacks opportunities that most whites took for granted (Myrdal, 1944). God might not be an American, exhorted preachers, but in God we could trust with confidence.

Members of the Great Generation taught their children to accept this version of the nation's Manifest Destiny. Focusing on domestic concerns and national priorities, they left it to the military, diplomats, and intelligence experts to do what they must overseas to preserve the American way of life. Unprecedented prosperity would enable a rising generation to do good and to do well. They could satisfy their personal aspirations while remedying domestic inequities, thereby setting an example for the world to admire.

A happy combination of economic and social circumstances, coupled with great expectations, made those born between 1946 and 1964 the "Lucky Generation" on several counts. Most parents invested time and money in their upbringing and schooling. The baby boomers were challenged to dream boldly as they matured. As youth, many supported the civil rights demands of African Americans and other disenfranchised groups. The Lucky Generation was the first cohort to feel the effects of a gender revolution that transformed professional schools, jobs, and bedrooms. But they had to learn the hard way that the world had become too interdependent for any single polity to dominate. "Far from this being a world of 'discrete civilisations' or simply an international order of states, it has become a fundamentally interconnected global order, marked by intense patterns of exchange as well as by clear patterns of power, hierarchy and unevenness" (Held, 1999: 49; see also Ignatieff, 2004).

The war in Vietnam marked a turning point in the boomers' learning curve. Thousands lost their lives; thousands more on their return home lost the will and ability to live normal lives. Baby boomers protested the arrogance of U.S. leaders for wasting capital, human and otherwise, in a civil war in a remote corner of the earth. The international community deplored the American folly. The debacle challenged prevailing assumptions about U.S. foreign policy. It provoked a distrust of government but did not fundamentally alter this cohort's sense of its place in the world order. Most baby boomers wanted to put the war behind them as fast as possible and get on with their lives. They had difficulty responding to humans' propensity for evil—the horrors of genocide in Africa, Asia, and South America, and brutal ethnic fighting in Europe. They still have trouble reaching out to victims of poverty, disease, and famine (Behrman, 2004; Griswold, 2004).

The end of the Cold War did not abrogate the responsibilities of the baby boom generation to respect the dignity of individuals at home and abroad. Indeed, they and the aging Great Generation must deal with global issues that did not concern their forbears. Two examples will suffice. The Club of Rome's *Limits to Growth* (1972) was a catalyst to global environmental politics comparable to the impact that Rachel Carson's *Silent Spring* (1964) had on American readers. Innumerable scientific reports and subsequent international conferences have documented the depletion of the earth's ozone layer, the destruction of tropical forests, and global warming. Thus far, transregional and transnational nongovernmental organizations have been the chief respondents to environmental crises. Although Americans of all ages have joined ecological groups ranging from saving whales to conserving woodlands, U.S. business and political leaders have by and large resisted commitments that might affect their businesses (Porter and Brown, 1991; Muller, 2002).

Second, 9/11 has become a red-letter date like December 7. The attack on the World Trade Towers and the Pentagon marked the first time that so many innocent Americans had lost their lives because they worked in buildings that symbolized U.S. financial and military might. An ignorance of world history has hampered the boomers' ability to respond to depravity. We know that fanatical fundamentalists orchestrated 9/11, yet our response thus far has led to debatable actions. Officials falsely linked the atrocity to a few nation states. Security measures taken by the U.S. government heightened fears and anxiety. Our foray into Iraq proved costly, financially and otherwise (Byrd, 2004; Committee on the Present Danger, 2004: A9). Yet another generation of Americans has proved itself to be oblivious to the risks of acting unilaterally in addressing interdependent global problems.

It is not too late for senior citizens to become exemplars of global responsibility. Against other terrifying threats to breath and life, dealing with the specter of global aging might not seem an obvious place to start. And given the reluctance of many citizens to think seriously about population aging in the United States, how great a constituency would be enticed to compare responses to demographic trends here and abroad? Yet population aging demands attention because of its effect on the marketplace, healthcare arena, and intergenerational relationships (among other things).

Although every nation is experiencing population aging, the demographic phenomenon varies from region to region. Nearly one-quarter of all people living in western European nations will be over 65 by 2030; it will remain the oldest region on earth. The United States, Canada, and Australia are not, and will not be, far behind. There will be a commensurate slowing of the growth of the working-age population in these countries, which probably will result in a continuation of outsourcing unskilled jobs to developing countries. There also will be competition for immigrants with specialized skills needed for countries to remain productive (Geipel, 2003; Greenspan, 2003).

Surprisingly, despite the comparatively higher fertility rates in the Third World, the elderly population is actually growing most rapidly south of the Equator. Developing nations have in their ranks roughly 59 percent of the world's senior citizens; that proportion is projected to rise to 71 percent by 2030. The oldest-old segment is the fastest-growing portion of the aging population in both developing and developed nations.

Demographers keenly monitor trends in Asia. Japan, which currently has the largest proportion of men and women over 65, expects one-third of its population to be elderly by 2030 (Bengtson and Lowenstein, 2003: 2–3, 6). In contrast to Western countries, where higher standards of living are associated with longevity, Japanese people with less education tend on average to outlive their better-educated peers (Liang et al., 2002: S294). Thanks to policies limiting couples to one child, the median age in China will rise from 32 today to 44 in 2040 (Kahn, 2004). This should enable the world's most populous nation to sustain short-term economic growth. However, some forecasters see dire times ahead as the proportion of people over 65 rises to 20 percent by 2015, because China has no effective pension programs (Asia, Inc., 1994: 3).

In discussing the economic implications of global aging, doomsayers have thus far dominated the dialog. "The costs of this global aging will probably be beyond the means of even the world's wealthiest nations, even if current retirement benefit systems are drastically reformed," asserts PriceWaterhouseCooper's London-based John Hawksworth (2002). "The problems engendered by this aged population will not only dominate the public policy agendas of the developed world, but will fundamentally alter the geopolitical order of the planet." Others agree that the widening imbalance between superannuated and productive workers threatens global economies, fundamentally altering the cultures of nation states (*Healthy Senior,* 2002; AARP, 2003b, 2003c). Taking a page from Americans for Generational Equity, some commentators envision a clash of generations over the demands of young people in developing countries and the needs of increasingly older cohorts in developed nations (Rothkopf, 2004).

With sufficient planning, however, optimists claim that the dire consequences of population aging can be averted. Canada, for instance, has been preparing its institutional network for increasing numbers of older people. Its public pension system is better funded than those elsewhere. Despite criticisms of access to its healthcare system, Canadian officials are sanguine about their ability to treat larger numbers of older men and women enjoying healthy, prosperous lives (Crane, 2004). Significant progress has been made to ensure that indigenous peoples have access to basic services. Boosts in productivity and increased volunteerism, anticipate experts, will provide a sufficient counterbalance to the costs of caring for the very old (Hart, 2001; Geipel, 2003: 4).

The inevitability and magnitude of population aging require seeing the interconnectedness of demography to other global priorities. AARP was one of the first age-based organizations to address the variety of challenges and opportunities associated with societal aging in a worldwide context. Since 1958 it has been a major source of information about demographic trends. Its officers brief foreign dignitaries as well as domestic leaders. AARP has also formed advocacy partnerships with the U.S. Council on Foreign Relations, the European Older People's Platform, and various units within the United Nations (AARP, 2003b, 2004).

Three other U.S. efforts illustrate the variety of global interests and initiatives. In 1999 Richard Estes, a University of Pennsylvania professor, created an archive that he called PRAXIS, a homepage aimed at social workers interested in promoting change in caring for aged people through social development (Estes, 2004). That same year the Center for Strategic and International Studies launched its Global Aging Initiative, an educational program dealing with what it deems the generally gloomy economic, social, and cultural consequences of population aging. Because of the organization's prestige, its publications have received extensive coverage in the transatlantic community and have served as the basis for Senate hearings and conferences in Europe and Japan (CSIS, 2004). In contrast, the International Center for Longevity, founded in 1990 by former National Institute on Aging director Robert N. Butler and Japanese colleagues, takes a more positive approach to the study of population aging. Its studies emphasize older people's productivity and the contributions that longer-lived individuals can make to their families and communities (International Longevity Center, 2004).

Other nations have sponsored landmark conferences and initiatives dealing with population aging. At the Fourth World Conference for Women in Beijing (1995), an Older Women's Tent was pitched. Roughly 1,500 women attending the conference indicated that "aging" was their first priority. On the last day of the conference, the women organized a network designed to concentrate on elder rights, economic security, and civic engagement through the auspices of nongovernmental organizations such as AARP, the China National Committee on Aging, HelpAge International, and Global Action on Aging (Paul, 1995).

To observe the U.N.-sponsored International Year of Volunteers (2001), the Council of Europe called on its constituent members to make unemployed elders more attractive to employers. It developed voluntary programs through which senior citizens could share their life experiences with the young. Besides encouraging the formation of partnerships among elderly people, refugees, migrants, and political leaders, the council emphasized the importance of using older professional volunteers in fields ranging from conflict resolution, the environment, and urban renewal. The initiatives depended on the cooperation of several dozen European groups already in place—not new organizations—to empower the continent's older men and women (Vincent, 1999; European Social Welfare Information Network, 1999; United Nations, 2000; Council of Europe, 2000: 2–3, 5).

One other tack merits notice: Japan has tapped the wisdom of its elders to complement the expertise of its public officials and private consultants in designing a plan to deal with societal aging. Senior citizens, mainstays of Japanese politics since the end of World War II, welcome opportunities to engage in the policymaking process, even if their tasks consist of simply staffing events, distributing materials, and mobilizing other elders (Economic Council, 1983). Here as elsewhere, customs are changing. Once the Liberal Democratic Party (LDP) could count on the support of senior citizens in return for social and healthcare services. But the LDP is losing ground as the number of nonaffiliated voters in urban areas increases; senior citizens must compete for support with those in straitened economic circumstances. As a result, Japan's aged people seek new allies and novel ways to contribute to the nation's productivity by returning to full-time employment, working part-time, or volunteering in the welfare arena (AARP, 2003c; Asahi.com, 2004).

Transnational bodies advocate for older people around the world. The International Federation on Ageing (IFA), founded in 1973, relies on older volunteers to exchange ideas, communicate concerns, and develop plans for the future. Based in Montreal, IFA currently links 151 associations in 54 nations. Declarations from its biennial conferences during the past two decades have often served as the basis for initiatives by the United Nations (International Federation on Ageing, 1999). Arguably a landmark in the history of global aging was the 1982 World Assembly on Aging, at which 183 nations were represented. Under the auspices of the United Nations, an International Plan of Action was formulated (Butler, 1998). In 1991, the U.N. General Assembly promulgated Principles for Older Persons. Four years later, the U.N. created an "architecture" for "a society of all ages," which emphasized new ways of valuing population aging and preparing youth, middle-aged, and older persons for the longevity revolution that is transforming their life courses (United Nations, 2003). The United Nations has also collaborated with the International Association of Gerontology and the Brookings Institution in preparing research agenda for population aging and implementing strategies to transform public management globally (Kettl, 2000; International Association of Gerontology, 2003).

Amid this array of national, regional, and global initiatives, we should not lose sight of efforts by independent senior citizens (often in developing nations) to enhance their well-being. Widows in a remote Indian village organized to appeal for aid in improving their circumstances. An 84-year-old grandfather in Kenya took advantage of a government reform that permitted him to attend grade school. For others, technology plays a critical role. The Internet enables a 67-year-old woman in India to keep in touch with daughters living in the United States. Senior citizens in rural Spain rely on the Internet, videos and CDs, and radios to upgrade their education and acquire skills so that they can reclaim their jobs. Robots offer therapy to victims of dementia in Japan; robots also are used there so human resources can be better deployed in social services (Pavon Rabasco et al., 2001; Global Action on Aging, 2004: 13–14, 18; Solidarity, 2004).

Senior citizens in developing countries who participate politically serve as role models for civic engagement throughout the world. Sometimes an exemplary individual or pair of activists demand justice in ways that attract international attention. Veerbala Nagarwadia, aged 91, has spent the last quarter-century fighting for the right of destitute elders to take refuge in nursing homes (Global Action on Aging, 2004: 2). Followers of two elderly Hanoi ministers mobilized to permit religious organizations besides the Buddhist Church of Vietnam to exist (Mercury News, 2003). A pair of older women in Belgrade used the Internet to mobilize opposition to the U.S. engagement in Bosnia (Activists Online, 1999). Senior citizens in Korea demanded the unconditional release of 17 sick prisoners who have been in solitary confinement for 28 to 40 years because of their imputed communist affiliations (Amnesty International, 1998). Senior citizens in China, who felt overlooked for the past two decades, developed an agenda to afford them more entertainment and volunteer activities; they also called for greater representation on municipal assemblies and urban councils (Chinese Century, 2001). Survivors exclusively serve as docents at the Holocaust Museum in Melbourne, Australia (Lehrman, 2002).

In and of themselves, these appear to be isolated instances. Yet they represent a harbinger of things to come: as leaders and followers, senior citizens have the passion and ability to promote justice and peace if moved to action. The lost lessons of the past, if recovered through the wisdom of experience, impel elders to act. U.S. senior citizens have prototypes to emulate.

Senior Citizens and U.S. Domestic Politics and Policy-Making

Incrementalism—augmenting programs policy amendment by policy amendment—has until lately shaped the politics of aging in the United States. Individuals, families, neighbors, and, in some instances, states, historically were responsible for caring for elderly men and women who could not maintain their independence. Except for Union veterans of the Civil War and those who joined the Townsend movement, senior citizens did not engage in collective action to benefit themselves or to help others in need. The political landscape changed when the federal government enacted old-age insurance and old-age assistance programs through the Social Security Act in 1935 (Brown, 1977). Thereafter, politicians, policy experts, and elderly people and their advocates lobbied for disability and healthcare coverage and for the expansion of social services and medical care. Washington was the hub of activity. Congress underwrote several national gatherings to develop an agenda to serve and empower senior citizens. Out of the 1961 White House Conference on Aging, for instance, came the blueprint for Medicare, Medicaid, and the Older Americans Act. The 1971 conferees did the spadework for consolidating various welfare agencies into the Supplemental Security Income program and dramatically liberalizing Social Security (Achenbaum, 1986; Berkowitz, 1991).

The federal government did not act alone. A gray lobby emerged. The first wave was dominated by charismatic figures such as Francis Townsend. The second consisted mainly of Mom-and-Pop organizations catering to segments of the aged population. During the 1960s, old-age interest groups grew in number and became more sophisticated in advocating for their memberships. There are now one hundred such organizations based in Washington (Pratt, 1976, 1993). To this must be added the various Area Agencies on Aging, instituted when President Richard Nixon in 1974 devolved to states the responsibility for delivering services. Experts in think tanks in universities and the private sector grappled with the purposes, mechanisms, and likely outcomes of legislation proposed by Congress, old-age organizations, and other interested parties. The collaborative efforts have paid off, even when the political climate was not conducive for constructive action. George W. Bush's administration has opposed national and international efforts to clean the environment, yet his Environmental Protection Agency in 2002 created a Web site to prioritize environmental health hazards; it encouraged senior citizens to become volunteers in their communities to promote health by reducing ecological risks (an initiative resembling a recommendation by the National Conference of Catholic Bishops). Addressing the needs of older Americans, as incrementalists had claimed for decades, ultimately benefited all age groups (National Conference of Catholic Bishops, 2001; Millett, 2003).

By the early 1980s, however, changes in the political economy, images of aging, and public philosophies began to undermine the effectiveness of the politics of incrementalism. Conservatives in business and government succeeded in persuading the public that the national government had to downsize. Because a large portion of the federal budget directly or indirectly went to senior citizens, old-age programs such as Social

Security became victims of their own success (Hudson, 1978). The 1983 amendments, while reaffirming the original purposes of the act, raised taxes and cut future benefits to ensure adequate retirement funds for the baby boom cohort (Achenbaum, 1986). The measure, hailed as a triumph of bipartisan negotiation, did not long succeed in allaying fears about Social Security's fiscal integrity. President George W. Bush, for instance, tenaciously advocates the program's privatization to avert a debatable fiscal "crisis."

The fate of the Medicare Catastrophic Coverage Act (MCCA) of 1988, moreover, revealed partisan and class divisions within the older population. MCCA was intended to cut the costs incurred during a major health crisis. In an era of fiscal austerity, these benefits were to be paid by Medicare recipients—and therein lay the rub. Affluent members of the aged cohort, who already had coverage through private insurance, did not want to support their less-fortunate peers. (Various measures of inequality indicate that the disparity in assets is greater within the population over 65 than among younger cohorts [Hendricks et al., 1999: 27].) Senior citizens bombarded Congress with petitions, pointing out flaws in the legislation. Some individuals physically attacked the act's architects. Stunned by the fallout, Congress repealed MCCA a year later. In fact, Congress wondered whether the gray lobby could fulfill its promises to rally constituents (Binstock and Quadagno, 2001).

Academics noted that the public and private institutions that served elderly people had not adapted to new political realities. Tactical and structural gaps in the infrastructure have become apparent. The 51-member Washington-based Leadership Council on Aging Organizations has "settled for talking to ourselves more than risked engagement with those who espouse different ideas or different interests," says Rother (2004: 56). Advocates who brilliantly championed the causes of the aged population in the 1970s have left the scene. Many member organizations of the gray lobby face internal problems—stagnant membership and shaky finances.

The political context has changed. The prevailing neoconservative ideology has shifted responsibility from the federal level to the states and private sector. It once sufficed to document the vicissitudes of late life to members of Congress, who in turn would broaden federal programs to lift a majority of elders above the poverty line. Now, more effort must be done at the grassroots level to secure legislative changes.

Even then, rather than celebrate victories that improve the lot of elderly people, pundits urged "greedy geezers" to forego entitlements. Individual sacrifices for the sake of the commonweal, conservatives claimed, would reduce the economic burdens associated with population aging (Hendricks et al., 1999: 28; Chapman, 2003; Peterson, 1999).

Furthermore, existing regulations often do not take account of the changing needs of various segments of the elderly population. The federal government's primary responsibility is to keep Social Security, the cornerstone of retirement in the United States, solvent. But Social Security is more than a public program; it greatly affects decision making in the private sector. Employers and employees make plans, assuming that the government pensions they expect to receive upon retirement actually will be there. Since the 1980s, a "crisis of confidence" has undermined workers' expectations concerning Social Security's long-term fiscal health. Thus far, few commentators have tried to sway public opinion concerning the relationship between Social Security's well-being and the financial health of corporate pensions. Yet regulatory changes in the former influence the latter.

The federal government monitors a variety of pension programs in the private sector. It oversees the Self-Employed Individuals Tax Retirement Act of 1962, sometimes called Keogh Plans. It also protects the investments workers make into corporate pensions under the Employee Retirement Income Security Act (ERISA) of 1974. Private pension coverage has neither been as uniform nor as universal as obtains under Social Security. Small firms just starting up, for instance, rarely create pension plans for their staffs. Moreover, there has been considerable disagreement among actuaries concerning what constitutes sufficient funding of private plans. Fiduciary standards governing corporate pensions are stricter than those that exist in most state and local plans, but a desire to reduce corporate tax liabilities often affects how and how much companies actually are willing to set aside (Achenbaum, 1986: 149–86; Walsh, 2004b, 2004c).

Then there is the specter of bankruptcy. The Enron fiasco appallingly illustrates the cost to workers. Many employees put all of their retirement funds in Enron's rising stock, confident that their company would continue to grow. When the bubble burst, they ended up with nothing. Unlike Enron's senior executives, workers could not remove their contributions as stock prices fell (Rapoport and Dharan, 2004). Enron is not an exceptional case. The future Social Security "crisis" pales in comparison to the losses currently experienced or anticipated in the private sector and for state and municipal employees (Walsh, 2004a). Bankrupt companies dumped $11 billion in obligations on the Pension Benefit Guaranty Corporation, leaving the agency with a growing deficit (*New York Times*, 2004). Taxpayers face even greater bills if airlines default on their pension commitments. The problems besetting Medicare and Medicaid are even more daunting.

Meanwhile the gender gap in federal programs, long recognized in Social Security, has not closed. Eligibility criteria still adversely affect older women. "The mismatch of current reality and archaic structure can be particularly punishing toward women," observed Robert Binstock. "Divorced women suffer from disadvantage in a system premised on the idea of life-time marriages. . . . Women who survive their spouses are also left vulnerable to impoverishment by antiquated Social Security rules" (Institute for Research on Women and Gender, 2002: 12).

Finally, experts ponder who *really* speaks for the elderly population's political interests at the national level. People join AARP to get discounts on prescriptions, travel, and other services. AARP tries to persuade advertisers that consumers over 50 represent a rich but relatively untapped market. But members rarely belong to AARP's local chapters or join its grassroots activities to mobilize support for legislative initiatives (Campbell and Skocpol, 2003: 2; Binstock, 2004). While the central office has latitude to operate as Washington insiders, critics charge that this does not really legitimize AARP's claim that in policy-making it speaks for its 35 million members. Social scientists contend that senior citizens are their own best representatives nationally. Seventy percent of men and women over 65 vote on a regular basis, twice the rate of people between 18 and 24. Senior citizens have the time to write letters, make phone calls from home, and perform a variety of voluntary tasks for causes that interest them—if they think their efforts will prove efficacious (Jennings and Markus, 1988; Day, 1990; Mulligan and Sala-i-Martin, 1999; Dychtwald, 2003a, 2003b).

The changing dynamics of the politics of aging in the United States became evident in the protracted fight to obtain prescription drug coverage under Medicare. The gray lobby claimed that sickly older people could not afford to pay for expensive medications. Polls indicated that almost two-thirds of all senior citizens supported this proposal; nine in ten wanted the federal government to negotiate lower prices with drug companies (Campbell and Skocpol, 2003). The media gave the issue coverage—though CBS was criticized for interviewing the same seven elderly activists on at least twenty-three occasions (Morano, 2003). Lawmakers expected the measure that Congress passed to reduce pharmacy bills by 15 percent, especially aiding low-income beneficiaries. But the Republican-backed measure had large holes in the benefit structure. Insurance companies and private health plans were accorded greater control over the future of Medicare (Pear, 2003). Elders got less drug coverage than expected, while Big Business emerged as the real winner in setting prices.

AARP spent $7 million in ads endorsing Medicare reform. Hundreds of angry members vented on the organization's Web site; some burned their AARP cards (Noonan and Carmichael, 2003). Such protests were predictable. So why would the nation's largest old-age group, long known for its centrist stances, support such a conservative measure? Analysts cite two reasons. First, insofar as AARP relies more on commercial income than membership dues, it could not ignore potential profits. Second, AARP is projecting a "younger" image to appeal to those over the age of 45. "This is definitely not your grandparents' AARP" (ibid.: 42; see also Stolberg and Freudenheim, 2003). Acknowledging that the legislation did not go far enough, AARP vowed to lobby for bigger drug benefits and the containment of future price increases. It supported an "Access to Benefits Coalition" spearheaded by the National Council on the Aging (NCOA) and 70 partners to inform elders with low incomes of their rights (Pear, 2004; Van Ryzin, 2004). And AARP's vigorous opposition to the privatization of Social Security should restore most members' confidence in the organization's commitment to advocate for its constituency in particular and the nation's cross-generational compact in general.

Unlike some sectors of society, senior citizens are well represented on the national political scene. The nation has been well served by congressional elders committed to social justice and peace. Think of Robert C. Byrd, who has excoriated the second Bush administration's domestic and foreign policies (2004); Sam Ervin, who kept the Watergate hearings on track; and Wayne Morse and Ernest Hollings, the only two senators to vote against giving Lyndon Johnson a mandate to escalate the war in Vietnam. Tireless advocates such as Robert Ball and the late Arthur Flemming and Claude Pepper defended Social Security well into their eighties (Berkowitz, 2003). Chief Justice Earl Warren and Justices William Brennan and Byron White fought for civil liberties until their dying breath. The list goes on, including people like John Gardner, who, after holding a cabinet position and heading the Carnegie Corporation, founded Common Cause to serve the public.

What *is* needed are more senior citizens willing to set aside their selfish interests and speak with experience on the national issues of the day. To this end, NCOA has created a council of elders to provide feedback on the agency's programs and to identify broad issues to pursue. Although no one could replace Maggie Kuhn, senior citizens should vivify the Gray Panthers, "tribal elders [who] are concerned about the tribe's survival" (K. Fischer, 1998: 98; Bukov et al., 2002). Those who once led institutions large or small know how to identify and rectify structural gaps and ideological lacunae in the current aging policy network. The brunt of the work, however, will be done by senior citizens who are followers, willing to work for humanitarian and political causes in their communities.

"Think Globally, Act Locally"

Senior citizens make some of their most important political contributions in their local communities and their family networks. British cleric and community activist Kenneth Leech shares philosopher Alasdair MacIntyre's conviction that creating "networks of small groups of friends, local forms of community" sustains "the virtues and the vision of a human future . . . from such local knowledge and local struggles, connections can, indeed must, be made with wider issues" (1992: 92, 141; see also MacIntyre, 1981: 245). Bookstores and the media abound in success stories of older Americans who urge neighbors to vote and who draft petitions to improve the quality of life in their locale, often as a way to help children and adolescents acquire what they need to become productive citizens themselves (Fisher, 2003: 54, 63–64, 83, 106; MoveOn.org, 2004: 22, 74, 76, 84, 92; Toner, 2004).

Senior citizens often engage at the grassroots level to advance global priorities discussed earlier in this chapter. For instance, elders joined other concerned citizens in Grand Rapids, Michigan, to recommend ways to promote "radiant justice." They insisted on a bottom-up approach, starting with the school system. Senior citizens offered to instruct young students on how to think critically and act decisively for the cause of justice and peace (Radiant Justice, 2000; see also McManus, 1996: 253).

In large cities and conservative rural towns, senior citizens have organized peace demonstrations, most recently against the war in Iraq. Their protests incorporate lessons of the past to comprehend current events. Seeing how her brother and son suffered traumatic stress after serving in World War II and Vietnam, for instance, an octogenarian activist in Oregon declared that "it was imperative to do *something.*" What she really hoped to accomplish was to build connections in the community, even among those who disagreed with her politics (Antieau, 2004).

Environmental issues matter (Environmental League, 2002). Senior citizens have been at the forefront in trying to conserve water resources and wetlands, maintain open spaces, and shut down dirty power plants for the sake of future generations. Jane Jacobs, whose *Death and Life of Great American Cities* (1961) transformed urban planning in North America, at 88 published another jeremiad, *Dark Age Ahead* (2004), in which she claims that the decay of the infrastructure, if left unattended, will destroy the environment (Krauss, 2004).

Intergenerational activities have sprung up in virtually every community in the United States. Objectives have not changed much over time— some initiatives assist needy older people; in other instances, senior citizens mentor the truly vulnerable. Such programs have become better planned and implemented over time. Successful ventures like ones conducted by On Lok Senior Health in San Francisco entail a wide range of activities, including programs to (re)train staff members who work with young and old (Lewis, 2002). Generations United (2004a, 2004b) maintains the nation's largest database of profiles and contact information on hundreds of intergenerational programs.

Intergenerational collaboration faces its most stringent test in urban revitalization, for it requires satisfying stakeholders who espouse conflicting views about what they consider to be equitable, environmentally sound, and economically viable. Community development succeeds or fails because of the civic engagement of leaders and followers who can think broadly and focus on local issues. The history of Seattle's International District illustrates how multicultural groups can interact with public and private institutions to save a low-income neighborhood. Chinese,

Japanese, Filipinos, African Americans, Koreans, Vietnamese, Cambodians, and Laotians made their neighborhood vibrant, despite natural disasters, racism, and other manufactured threats (see especially International District, 2004; HistoryLink.org, 2004).

The Chinese came to Seattle first in the 1860s to build railroads, pave roads, and work in lumber mills and on fishing boats. By 1876, they constituted one-sixth of the city's population. The Chinese Exclusion Act (1882), however, halted further immigration; white settlers forcibly removed Chinese citizens from their homes. The Great Seattle Fire of 1889 destroyed what remained of Old Chinatown; streets were under water until the area was regraded in 1907. With the opening of Union Station four years later, Chinese entrepreneurs built hotels and businesses nearby.

The Japanese, who were not affected by restrictive immigration laws and who (unlike the Chinese) could bring their families to the United States, began to settle close to Old Chinatown. By 1910, Seattle's largest minority had built restaurants, laundries, and bathhouses; Dearborn Street, local mapmakers noted, was also known as Mikado Street. The Japanese community prospered until 1942, when Presidential Order 9066 relocated 7,000 residents to internment camps. In their absence, part of the original Japan Town was demolished to make way for the city's first public housing project. African Americans, lured by jobs with Boeing, settled in the area. The district then became the city's jazz center. (Ray Charles had his first gig in one of the district's hotels.)

Filipinos began to settle in Seattle shortly after the Japanese migrated; they worked primarily in farming and in the salmon/cannery industries. Unlike the Chinese and Japanese, the Filipinos protested their poor working conditions. Led by Carlos Bulosan (1911–56), Filipinos organized unions to rectify the discrimination they encountered. Bulosan's semi-autobiographical account of his labor activities, *America Is in the Heart* (1946), established him as one of the nation's premier Filipino authors (deLeon, 1999). By 1990, Filipinos constituted Seattle's largest minority population.

In the 1950s, the district was once again deteriorating: streets were dimly lit; many single homes were fire hazards. The construction of Interstate 5 and a stadium threatened to destroy the district. Mayor William Devin renamed the neighborhood "International Center" and pledged support to stem decay and to fight the segregation of Asian Americans.

The election of Wing Luke (1925–65) as the first Chinese American on Seattle's city council gave minority groups access to the city leaders. The end of immigration restrictions in 1965 opened gates to a growing number of Chinese from Hong Kong and southern provinces, Japanese, and Filipinos as well as Pacific Islanders. This infusion of new blood proved crucial to community revitalization.

Student activists, pledging Asian-American unity, lobbied for low-income housing, historic preservation, and bilingual social services. Professionals set up offices in buildings where their parents and grandparents had once lived (MacIntosh, 2003; Wing Luke Asian Museum, 2004). The establishment of the intramural Inter*Im Community Development Association in 1969 to benefit low-income and minority residents created the organizational framework for community action. Its leader, Filipino American Bob Santos (1934–), has mentored a generation of activists who now head neighborhood advocacy groups. Iter*Im helped to integrate new waves of immigrants—Vietnamese, Cambodians, and Laotians—into the district. "Uncle Bob" served seven years under the Clinton administration as Pacific Northwest director of the Department of Housing and Urban Development (HUD). Santos nonetheless views his chief accomplishment to be engaging nonactivists in the preservation of past traditions (Derr, 2002; Inter*Im, 2002; Preservation Seattle, 2002; Quintance, 2004).

Besides successfully negotiating with corporate executives and federal agencies, Bob Santos drew in residents of the district who were reluctant to get involved. He encouraged younger members of the Chinese-American community to capture the memories of a dying generation, who had been too humble and fearful of immigration authorities to speak out. The four-year project resulted in oral histories from seventy-one pioneers (Higgins, 1994). And while third- and fourth-generation children generally preferred to leave the International District for the suburbs, some longstanding groups, such as the Eng Family Association, hold social events, offer scholarships, and sponsor international meetings every four years (Higgins, 2004). The elders oversee these activities.

Revitalization continues, now assisted by HUD, Community Development Block Grants, and the Seattle Office of Economic Development. The district is an aging neighborhood: nearly a third of the residents are over 65; only a tenth are under the age of 16. Roughly three-fifths of the population have incomes below the poverty line. Unemployment exceeds

13 percent. Thus, the creation of low-income housing, a critical need since the 1930s and 1940s, remains a paramount priority. So does elder care. In the late 1990s, a 44,000-square-foot facility was created to house 75 frail elders; it also reaches 200 others who live in the neighborhood (Higgins, 1996; Preservation Seattle, 2002).

Ethnic rivalries flare occasionally. Some want the neighborhood to be called Chinatown/International District to reflect its origins; Japanese Americans feel that their community, Nihonmachi, was obscured in the historic preservation of the Pan-Asian area (Higgins, 1997; Charrette, 2003). Tensions arise from the demographic mix. Half the residents are foreign born: 56 percent are Asian or Pacific Islanders; 15 percent, African American and white, respectively; and 5 percent, Latino (Neighborhood Revitalization Strategies, 2002: Appendix B-1; International District, 2004). The International District is nonetheless a prime example of how marginalized people can (re)create interesting multicultural communities if they rely on the strengths of neighbors of all ages, preserve the best of the past, and create institutional support to address pressing needs (*Seattle-Post Intelligencer,* 2004).

In neighborhoods such as the International District, families function as little commonwealths all over America. Thanks to the longevity revolution, senior citizens and other intergenerational kin foster domestic cohesion. "In the narratives of social democracy, the aging family is seen as a reservoir of potential social inclusion" (Bengtson and Lowenstein, 2003: 109). Historical demographer Peter Uhlenberg calculates that children born in 1900 had an 18 percent chance of being orphaned before they reached their eighteenth birthday. U.S. children born a century later have a 68 percent chance that they will have four or more grandparents still alive in 2018; by the time they reach 30, three-quarters are expected to have at least one living grandparent. Co-survivorship across generations in an era of divorce, remarriage, and blended families makes possible a kin supply of (great)grandparents, aunts, and uncles to supplement parental support. Elders can bolster educational and social services in the community for children of all races and classes in need (ibid.: 10–11; Bengtson, Rosenthal, and Burton, 1995).

Population aging affects family dynamics in positive, negative, and paradoxical ways. One out of eight older persons cares directly for his or her grandchildren. Grandparents, according to one estimate, contribute the equivalent of between $17 and $29 billion annually in unpaid supervision and care for their grandchildren. Such support is critical, even heroic, when the parents are single, divorced, unemployed, imprisoned, or suffering from addiction, mental illness, disability, or AIDS (Butler, 1998: 3; Bengtson and Lowenstein, 2003: 76–77).

Some parents, however, resent their own parents' child-raising techniques. Sometimes they feel caught in the middle, obliged to assist at both ends of the life course. Caring for (widowed) grandparents who are in failing health and who live in isolation far away can, in turn, strain family emotions and resources. Families supply 60 to 80 percent of the initial care for dependent elders before turning to institutional facilities when the elders' decline becomes too physically and emotionally draining to handle. Female family members, who do most of the caregiving, sometimes feel divided loyalties at home and at work. Significant detachment or conflict affects roughly one-fifth of all eldercare relationships. Statistics estimating that 3 percent of all older Americans are abused by family members—more likely by spouses than by their children—probably underestimate the extent of the problem because of underreporting (McGinnis and McGinnis, 1984: 2; Pillemer and Finkelhor, 1988; Pillemer et al., 2000; Bengtson and Lowenstein, 2003: 13).

Contemporary researchers invoke at least two paradoxes about intergenerational ties within family networks. First, divorce dissolves more than marital bonds: the anger, hurt, and financial consequences of the break-up disrupts bonds of affection and potential sources of support between grandparents and grandchildren. While the fabled wicked stepmother sometimes has counterparts in the third and fourth generations, there is evidence that many cross-generational links remain intact. Second, although the duration and commitments made by gays and lesbians are often as enduring as those between married couples, states and religious organizations wrestle with how much recognition they wish to accord same-sex partnerships as family units. Grandparents have a stake in the outcome. Are they legally and financially bound to nurture the children their offspring adopt? Too often lost in the debate is the respect and rights due to senior citizens eager to share their love and poised to intervene when necessary.

The love, wisdom, and care given by grandmothers and grandfathers make for inspiring stories (Fays, 2002). And the tug at the heartstrings has commercial value. Marian Lucille Herndon McQuade proposed in 1970 that a special day be set aside for grandparents, comparable to the celebrations of Mother's and Father's days. McQuade was a West Virginia housewife with fifteen children, forty grandchildren, and eight great-grandchildren. As president of the Vocational Rehabilitation Foundation, she knew how to get legislation passed. After three years of lobbying, McQuade persuaded West Virginia to establish the first Grandparents Day. In 1978 President Jimmy Carter proclaimed National Grandparents Day to be the first Sunday after Labor Day, a time to honor life's "autumn years" (National Grandparents Day, 2004). The holiday increasingly is celebrated with cards, sweets, and intergenerational festivities. Organizations such as the Foster Grandparents Program and Generations United use the event, in Margaret Mead's words, "to restore a sense of community, a knowledge of the past, and a sense of the future" (Generations United, 2004a).

More recently, senior citizens have organized to ensure, through legal mechanisms, their rights as grandparents and to protect their grandchildren. "Grandparents for Children's Rights" staged a rally in 2002 that quickly spawned forty-one chapters throughout the nation. A year later New York passed a law affecting 413,000 grandparents heading households in which grandchildren live, to keep together families at risk. The measure, which also strengthens visitation rights, has served as a model in other jurisdictions such as North Carolina. Under consideration in the Empire State is legislation that would give relatives supporting children a stipend equal to 75 percent of the foster care rate. The federal government is beginning to take action, in part because regulations and benefits vary so much at the state level. In 2004, noting a 30 percent increase in children living in grandparent-headed households and another 1.5 million children living with other relatives, Senator Hillary Rodham Clinton and fourteen colleagues introduced a bill that would promote policies that support grandparents' efforts to remove barriers to caregiving. The measure also recommended respite care, housing, and subsidized guardianship for grandparents and relatives raising children outside of foster care (U.S. Senate, 2004).

One final kinship matter must be addressed: families have to confront end-of-life issues, because sooner or later everybody dies. Most would prefer to succumb peacefully at home surrounded by their loved ones. However, data gathered over the past decade indicate that one in four Americans dies suddenly; half are conscious enough to suffer at least moderate pain during their final days, and at least one-third spend the last ten days of their lives in an intensive-care unit (Potter, 1998: 5; APA,

2001b). Minorities, persons with dementia, and people over 80 are more likely than others to have their pain untreated, their physicians unaware of their preferences (Byock, 1999).

As the U.S. population ages, death increasingly occurs in late life. As noted in chapter 1, seven out of ten Americans die past the age of 65, roughly one-quarter of these after 85 (Hobbs and Damon, 1996: 3–4). More than one-third of all Medicare dollars are allocated to older persons in the terminal stages of life. In this context, the management of dying and death is the ultimate act of senior citizenship. Debates currently under way over elders' rights and responsibilities as they lie dying will have a profound impact on how we grapple with ethical, social, and fiscal issues in an aging society. Nowhere is the personal so political, or vice versa.

Fortunately, individuals and institutions have taken steps to relieve the fear and pain associated with dying. Since the establishment of a hospice in New Haven in 1974, increasing numbers of healthcare centers have followed suit. Hospice, specifically created to help persons at the end of life, has extended its reach through Medicare funding. Once offered only in homes and designated settings, hospices now cooperate with nursing homes with good results (Quality of Life Matters, 2002). Hospice principles and practices have now been applied in other settings under the rubric of palliative care. While some distinguish between the two modalities—the latter often begins earlier treatment of a life-threatening but not necessarily fatal disease—the common features outweigh the differences (Byock, 1998). According to Christine Cassel, "palliative care [affords] broad and integrated physical, psychological, social, and spiritual care for patients with serious diseases that might be life threatening" (Milbank, 2000: 4). Hospice caregivers and palliative care specialists work along an interdisciplinary continuum.

Leading U.S. hospitals, such as Massachusetts General and Memorial Sloan-Kettering, have established palliative care programs. Whereas only 1 percent of all medical facilities in 1983 had multidisciplinary ethics teams to evaluate difficult cases, within a decade more than three-fifths of all hospitals had formed such bodies (APA, 2001a, 2003a). Coalitions to support good-quality care in late life have sprung up (Aging with Dignity, 2004; Compassion in Dying Federation, 2004; Last Acts Partnership, 2004). Clergy and faith communities minister to the dying through Stephen's Ministries, parish nurses, and Communities of Hope (Byock, 1999; Catholic Apologetics, 2004; Malley, 2004).

In the wake of the Patient Self-Determination Act of 1991, the legal community has created instruments to ensure good-quality care. One-quarter of all Americans have living wills that specify the care they wish when they become terminally ill or incapacitated. With a durable power of attorney for health care, an individual can assign a surrogate to make decisions—though the usefulness of this document has been challenged on grounds that people tend to change their minds about treatment when they are face-to-face with death (Hagelberg, 1997; Morrison, 2000; APA, 2003b; Gearon, 2003). Local, state, and federal officials have joined the end-of-life bandwagon. "Clearly a political leadership exists that has found end-of-life care a positive issue with virtually no political downside, because every single constituent in these leaders' districts benefits from good end-of-life care policy" (State Initiatives, 2001).

Yet some end-of-life issues divide politicians and electorate. The Hemlock Society, founded in 1980 and now called End-of-Life Choices, supports the right of persons with a terminal disease (not just hopelessly ill) to commit suicide. It distributes a how-to-do-it guide called *Final Exit* (Goodenough, 2003; *Washington Post*, 2003: A07; Friedman, 2004). Although the Supreme Court in two 1997 cases, *Vacco v. Quill* and *Washington v. Glucksberg,* declared that there was no constitutional right to physician-assisted suicide, it permitted states to judge the matter. That same year Oregon passed a carefully crafted Death with Dignity Act, permitting the practice under stringent criteria. A 1999 federal bill would have extended training in palliative care, but it also would have voided the Oregon law. Supported by the American Medical Association and the National Hospice Association and opposed by the American Pharmaceutical Association, the bill languished in Congress (APA, 2003c: 2; www.oregonline).

Medical ethicists and philosophers fiercely debate euthanasia and physician-assisted suicide. Norman Daniels (1988) and Jane English (1993) question whether children are morally obliged to care for their aged parents, emphasizing the principle of individual autonomy in exercising their right to die. Daniel Callahan advocates research that would prevent premature deaths, but he sees no societal value in prolonging useless existence. The Hastings Center, the organization he founded, published a guideline with practical advice to complement his position (Hastings Center, 1987; D. Callahan, 2003). In contrast to Jack Kevorkian's arbitrary criteria for assisting 130 people who sought his help to die, Timothy Quill offers a sobering observation: "If we are to extend ourselves as a compassionate society to openly sanction physician-assisted suicide as the intervention of last resort, we must not allow our ambivalence about the act to let us ignore the circumstances when it does not work" (1996: 176).

Opponents question whether everyone possesses the same resources to exercise individual autonomy in making decisions. Some lack the financial wherewithal, critical acumen, and medical information to make an informed decision. Religious beliefs preclude others from contemplating suicide. Ethnic groups differ. African Americans and Hispanics are more likely than whites to opt for life-sustaining support. Mexican and Korean immigrants may put more emphasis on family solidarity than autonomy. Chinese families tend to protect the dying from negative information. Other cultures hold that talking about dying is an invitation to death (APA, 2003c, 2003d). Sidney Callahan joins feminists in opposing euthanasia: "Feminist ideals of inclusive justice, caretaking, and interconnectedness of all the living require that we struggle against approving assisted suicide and euthanasia. Let there be no more recruits for the armies of domination and death" (2004: 9; see also Chavez, 1999; APA, 2003b, 2003c).

In my opinion, the case against euthanasia complements the aims of an aging society. Individual autonomy is to be valued, but it must be exercised in the context of interconnecting elements of our diverse population. Contingencies and exigencies make our lives as fragile as the institutions and relationships we create. The mysteries of death and dying attest to the transitory nature of the human condition. With sufficient palliative mechanisms to treat the terminally ill with dignity, there are lessons to share and embrace at the final moment. As T. S. Eliot concluded "East Coker" in his *Four Quartets* (1952: 129):

> Home is where one starts from. As we grow older
> The world becomes stranger, the pattern more complicated. . . .
> Old men ought to be explorers
> Here and there does not matter.

Life's uncertain journey makes us all explorers. It does not, in the final analysis, matter where and how senior citizens teach us to share or to grow. The opportunity to contribute is a gift, not just an obligation of extra years.

{ Epilogue

No single man or woman could embody the major themes just explored, but Mungo and Abayah Martin come close. The age-old indigenous way of life in British Columbia into which they were born in the late nineteenth century was collapsing. The Martins survived long enough, however, to play instrumental roles in late life in preserving, promoting, and extending the traditional culture and tribal arts they learned in youth.

Mungo Martin was born in 1879, one of four sons of a ranking figure among the Kwakiutl people. His father died when Mungo was a boy. His mother then married Charlie James, one of the renowned carvers in the community. Mungo apprenticed with his stepfather, thus fulfilling his mother's wish that this son be given the magic to create totem poles and other pieces of Northwest Coastal art. Abayah was born in 1890. As a child she mastered all of the skills appropriate for women: she knew how to make cedar bark clothing and baskets and to weave and embroider blankets. Married first to David Hunt, another master of Kwakiutl art, she then wed Mungo Martin. Together they endeavored to recollect ceremonial lore and customs, to recall ritual songs, and to remember the techniques of the various crafts they mastered (A. Hawthorn, 1979: 257–58).

Mungo and Abayah's commitment to carrying on historical memory was critical, because their culture slowly was being destroyed by forces beyond their control. At first the Hudson Bay Company's trading posts at Fort Langley, Fort Victoria, and Fort Rupert (established between 1827 and 1845) benefited the indigenous tribes: the Kwakiutl could sell their carvings and crafts as well as acquire goods for potlatching—elaborate feasts in which gifts were exchanged to attest to the prestige and influence of various ruling families. However, from 1838 until its peak in 1862, disease decimated villages, leaving 20,000 dead. A later cohort of tribal people abandoned their homesteads when smallpox and an influenza epidemic struck in 1918. "Old houses were decaying along deserted village sites, facing the sea. Inheritance of great houses, with traditional names and with appropriate crest poles and house posts, seemed to be disappearing, as families coped with the post depression economic adjustment to a national society with new standards" (ibid.: vii; B.C. Indian Arts Society, 1982: 8).

Disease was not the only threat to the vitality of Kwakiutl culture. British officials treated the northwest tribes as a subjugated group in an obscure corner of their empire. The Kwakiutl were forced to comply with imperial mandates, including the government ban on potlatching in 1884. Missionaries felt that pagan rituals hindered their efforts to convert indigenous people to Christianity. Public officials feared that the esteem accorded native rulers would undercut the Crown's authority. Since the Kwakiutl viewed the potlatch as a substitute for intertribal warfare, its curtailment had diplomatic as well as social ramifications (B.C. Indian Arts Society, 1982: 7). There were a few instances of surreptitious potlatches occurring on the northwest coast during the prohibition, but the infrequency of the ceremony and modest array of gift giving were signs that a proud culture was being dismantled by outside administrative control.

Some tried to live in two worlds. Chief Mungo Martin adapted to white man's world by becoming a commercial fisherman; his boat had a motorized engine. He occasionally carved totem poles, which the Royal Mounted Canadian Police confiscated. Abayah stayed home, crocheting and weaving. The couple persevered in remembering the wisdom and artistic techniques of their elders. They could not imagine doing otherwise. The Martins felt that the spirit of their community was fragile; it was atrophying as they grew older.

In 1947 an opportunity to give new life to northwestern coastal art presented itself. The University of British Columbia's Department of Anthropology invited Mungo Martin, then 67, to come to campus.

They wanted Chief Martin to restore some totem polls and carve some new ones for their collection, which had begun twenty years earlier with the acquisition to two house posts from another tribe. Mungo leapt at the chance. He saw the museum as a suitable site for preserving the treasures of his culture. The chief proved to be a productive carver. Working eight-hour days, he first created two 40-foot poles for the British Columbia Museum of Anthropology and then accepted commissions elsewhere. (One pole, crafted for Queen Elizabeth II, stands in London's Windsor Park.) Bored during a brief hospitalization, Mungo began to draw crest paintings in the native colors of green, red, and black. He narrated to students the symbolism embodied in the details of his art. Abayah accompanied her husband to the University of British Columbia, where she wove and taught others to weave blankets and aprons.

In late life Mungo and Abayah did whatever they could to revitalize their culture. They spoke extensively with anthropologist Franz Boas, who recorded their ethnographies. Mungo advised the Department of Anthropology concerning what artifacts to buy for their collection of Northwest Coastal art. When the British lifted the ban on potlatches in 1951, the Martins were instrumental in instructing young people about the appropriate sequence of rituals, the range of musical chants, and the politics of gift-giving. One of the first potlatches Chief Martin orchestrated was to "open the house," a large Kwakiutl structure near the museum (Jonaitis, 1991: 57; A. Hawthorn, 1979: 257–58). Both Abayah and Mungo taught younger people who wanted to learn traditional Kwakiutl crafts and carving. As mentors they urged their apprentices to be faithful to tradition but not bound by it. The Martins wanted the rising generation of artists to adapt classic symbols and styles, applying their own imaginations and aesthetic sensibilities. Abayah and Mungo believed that Kwakiutl culture could flourish once again if and when a critical mass of artists developed their own idiom. By now a living icon, Chief Martin was invited to represent his people on various commissions and at hearings aimed at improving the welfare of coastal tribes.

Martin Mungo remained at the University of British Columbia until his death at 83; Abayah died shortly later. "No Canadian Indian did more than Chief Martin to secure recognition and honor for the cultures of his people," observed Frederica de Lagun (1963: 894–96) in a eulogy in the *American Anthropologist,* "and so helped to win for the Indians equal rights under Provincial and Federal Canadian laws."

The gift of extra years made it possible for Mungo and Abayah Martin late in life to share their creativity, memories, and energy to benefit two cultures. Longevity per se is a necessary, but not sufficient ingredient of this tale. The Martins had accumulated a lifetime of valuable experiences that they could pass on. Each kept in mind tribal customs and art-making learned in childhood and youth. They refined and adapted their skills through middle age, even in the face of opposition from Imperial powers. The fruits of their creative talent are amply displayed at the British Columbia Museum of Anthropology. Mungo and Abayah were generous with their time and wisdom. The students they mentored became the leaders of the second wave of coastal artists; and they, in turn, are now training the third and fourth cohorts. The Martins' legacy lives on through the commitment of young people to preserve a culture that disease, destruction, and disarray might have eliminated. By preserving the past in the face of obstacles, Mungo and Abayah were able, late in life, to infuse their culture with new spirit and vitality.

The Martins, of course, did not act alone. Their relationships with various institutions are integral to this story. Had the British Columbia Museum of Anthropology not wished to collect Kwakiutl art (and had Chief Martin decided he would not work with whites whose forebears ruined his way of life), there would be no story. Nor would the museum have been able to acquire two totems in 1927 without the financial backing of alumni, the university president, provincial government officials, B.C. Packers, Ltd., and Union Steamships (A. Hawthorn, 1979: vii). And whereas the Martins' influence was felt mainly on the coast of British Columbia, the contact with Franz Boas, a dean of anthropology, established an outlet to a larger audience interested in how indigenous societies develop identities through rituals and art.

This book offers ample proof that communities, local and global, have reaped innumerable benefits from men and women accorded extra years of living. It does not ignore risks associated with population aging, but treats them as comparable to other large-scale shifts in focus and locus of relationships, individual and institutional (Beck, 1992; Dodd, 1999). The grounds for optimism outweigh reasons for fearing economic crises and social dislocation because of societal aging. America's elders contribute the equivalent of $1 billion in volunteer services; some propose the creation of a "Boomer Corps" to attract more aging boomers into educating our youth (Gafni, 2003: 203; Dychtwald, 2003b; Butler, 1998: 3; New DemocratsOnline, 2004). The transformation of the meanings and experiences of old age, on balance positive, is already under way.

Acknowledging the untapped potentials and capacities among those over 70 affords individuals and institutions new choices in crafting novel lifestyles and roles of responsibility. The heterogeneity inherent in cohorts of individuated, longer-lived persons provides greater opportunities for interactions with different age groups and service to the broader community (Phillipson, 1998: 47; Gilleard and Higgs, 2000).

Although this book does not call for radical societal change, certain themes that recur require us to alter our perceptions, policies, and actions.

• *Myopia:* We can no longer deny the importance of population aging in thinking about our individual and collective futures. The percentages of men and women over 65 and over 80 are rising in both developing and developed countries. This means that nations have a new source of productivity at their disposal, one that is far too valuable (and expensive) to be discounted or discarded. Policymakers and ordinary citizens must take account of societal aging in planning for the future. We can make plans that work to our collective advantage. It is not enough to laud Mungo and Abayah Martin for sharing their creative gifts at advanced ages. We must also credit them for showing rising generations of artists how to adapt to institutions as they take advantage of organizational change.

• *Ageism:* More than economic fears, ageism animates our concern about individual and societal aging. We have not moved very far in extirpating the prejudice against older people since the 1960s when the term was coined. Surprisingly, despite the gains in adult longevity, "65" remains the point in the life course in which stereotypic, disparaging images of age become prominent and virulent. Myopia compounds the ageism because we do not distinguish sharply between personal and societal aging. Societal ageism pits the interests of one cohort against another instead of synergizing people at various stages of the life course. Such ageism is widespread in the marketplace, in the healthcare arena, in education institutions, and in religious circles. The prejudice, individual and institutional, feeds on itself: had Mungo and Abayah Martin not devoted their lives to preserving their culture, they would have had fewer lessons to impart, assuming anyone cared. Had provincial institutions not recognized the Martins as wise elders, the Kwakiutl way of life might have vanished.

• *Disconnected institutions and policies*: The compartmentalization of the human life course to three boxes of life—education, work, and retirement—has become obsolete. Age-graded institutional silos reduce the ability of men and women as they grow older to shift careers, to circle in and out of volunteer activities, to explore new ideas, and even to reinvent themselves. Although some elders prefer to withdraw, many older women and men prove quite successful in making existing institutions serve their ends. For most of their lives, Mungo and Abayah had to hide their heritage and conform to white people's expectations. They could not legally participate in potlatches because missionaries and provincial officials found them threatening. But options changed when the Martins were past the prime of life. Once the institutional context in which they lived altered dramatically, the chief and his wife responded accordingly. An academic museum joined forces with government units and local companies to preserve a culture that was fading away. It was a vision—the importance of preserving an indigenous way of life—that gave institutions a mission and in the process afforded the Martins a critical role in its fulfillment.

• *Spirituality looks outward, not just inward:* Theologians and gerontologists have told us much about the spiritual dimension of late life at the individual level; its institutional components demand greater attention. This book offers many illustrations of how spiritual impulses motivate service to others within and beyond the religious realm. We saw this in senior citizens' activities in the healthcare arena, in mentoring and volunteering, in learning, and in intergenerational bonds in the public and private spheres. At bottom, the totem poles and carvings that Chief Martin crafted and the baskets and blankets Abayah Martin wove were *spiritual* creations: the symbols they designed were based on historical patterns; their art bore witness to the belief within the Kwakiutl northwest coastal tribe that animals connect humans to the divine, that transformations of the human spirit are frequent in nature. In maintaining these symbols, the Martins' legacy was to keep a tradition vibrant, capable of renewal.

The story of Mungo and Abayah Martin has counterparts around the world. The happy coincidences that surrounded their life histories are distinctive, not unique. Institutional forces and anonymous individuals made it possible for the Martins to embody vital aging. The contingencies and ironies of human existence cannot be overestimated. Tragedy and failure are part of mortals' fate. Still, Shakespeare gives us a measure of hope through the voice of an old man in one of his minor plays:

That nature's fragile vessel doth sustain
In life's uncertain voyage, I will some kindness do them.
(Timon of Athens, 5.1.206–7)

The human condition is fragile, enveloped by contingencies. Making one's way in "life's uncertain voyage" is fraught with danger. But Timon, a great lord reduced to miserable conditions at advanced age, understood the importance of kindness to fellow citizens and to humankind. With seniority comes a maturity that often (but not always) culminates in practical experience. The renewed-old in our midst, taking advantage of extra years of life, attain a wisdom by turns worldly and sublime. It ripens with experience and through fulfilling one's responsibility to show "kindness" to kin, to neighbors, and to strangers alike. Societal aging is generative insofar as it cultivates a "mature imagination" based on altruism. Societal aging requires organizational structures that nurture the capacity of senior citizens to utilize lessons from the past while joining young and middle-aged men and women in promoting justice and mercy in a world all too prone to endure violence and to tolerate suffering (Biggs, 1999; see also Gullette, 2004). In exercising their mature imagination, those at the forefront of societal aging are ideally positioned to tap their personal experiences for broader social purposes. Our challenge is to see the potential that comes with longevity. If we do so, we can tap virtues of extra years as we cope with the fragilities and uncertainties along our journeys through life.

REFERENCES

All URLs were accurate as of February 21, 2005.

AARP. 2003a. "AARP Names 'Best Employers for Workers over 50.'" *Business and Legal Reports.* www.newwork.com/Pages/NewsArchives/2003/Sept03 .html

———. 2003b. "The New Old World: Politics of Aging." September. www.aarp .org/international-events/Articles/a2003-10-10-politicspaneloverview.html

———. 2003c. "Japan 2003: The Politics of Aging." www.aarp.org/international/ Articles/a2003-09-25-Saidel.html

———. 2004. "AARP Global Aging Program." www.aarp.org/international/ Articles/a2002-08-01-aboutia.html

Abelson, Reed. 2003. "Fewer Retirees Get Drug Coverage from Employers." *New York Times,* July 23, C1.

Achenbaum, W. Andrew. 1978a. *Old Age in the New Land.* Baltimore: Johns Hopkins University Press.

———. 1978b. "From Womb through Bloom to Tomb." *Reviews in American History* 6:178–83.

———. 1986. *Social Security: Visions and Revisions.* New York: Cambridge University Press.

———. 1995a. "Age-Based Jewish and Christian Rituals." In *Aging, Spirituality, and Religion,* eds. Melvin A. Kimble et al. Minneapolis: Fortress Press.

———. 1995b. *Crossing Frontiers: Gerontology Emerges as a Science.* New York: Cambridge University Press.

———. 2004. "Wisdom's Vision of Relations." *Human Development* 47 (September–October): 300–303.

Achenbaum, W. Andrew, and Malcolm H. Morrison. 1993. "Is Unretirement

Unprecedented?" In *Achieving a Productive Society,* ed. Scott A. Bass, Francis G. Caro, and Yung-Ping Chen. Westport, Conn.: Auburn House.

Achenbaum, W. Andrew, Steven Weiland, and Carole Haber. 1996. *Keywords in Sociocultural Gerontology.* New York: Springer Publishing.

Activists Online. 1999. "Toward Freedom." www.towardfreedom.com/jul99/activistsonline.htm

Adams, James Truslow. 1944. *Frontiers of American Culture.* New York: Charles Scribner's Sons.

Adherents.com. 2002. "Largest Religious Groups in the United States of America." www.adherents.com/rel_USA.html

Adventist Development and Relief Agency. 2003. "Report." www.give.org/reports/care_dyn.asp?780

Agency for Healthcare Research and Quality. 2001. *Improving the Health and Health Care of Older Americans.* Washington, D.C.: U.S. Public Health Service.

Aging Today. 1998. "Mentors Pass Along Professional Legacy in Minority Aging."

Aging with Dignity. 2004. www.agingwithdignity.org

Alcoholics Anonymous. 2004. "Questions and Answers about Alcoholics Anonymous." www.alcoholics-anonymous.org/default/en_about_aa_sub.cfm?subpageid=55&pagei

Alliance for Aging Research. 2003. *Ageism: How Healthcare Fails the Elderly.* Washington, D.C.: Alliance for Aging Research.

———. 2004. *Redesigning Healthcare for an Aging Nation.* Washington, D.C.: Alliance for Aging Research.

American Association of Homes and Services for the Aging. 2002. "Restructuring Medicare." www.aahsa/org/member/commiss.htm

———. 2004. "Where AAHSA Stands on Long Term Care." www.aahsa.org/stand.htm

American Baptist Church. 1987. "American Baptist Resolution on Older Americans." www.abc-usa.org/resources/resol/older.htm

American Geriatrics Society. 1998. "Areas of Basic Competency for the Care of Older Patients for Medical and Osteopathic Schools." www.americangeriatrics.org/products/positionpapers/competency/shtml

American Jewish Communities. 2001. "Major National Jewish Organizations Come Together around Senior Long-Term Care Issues." www.uja.org/content_display.html?ArticleID=11488

American Journal of Public Health. 1998. "Religious Elderly Tend to Live Longer." www.personalmd.com/news/a1998100606.shtml

American Psychological Association (APA). 2001a. "End-of-life Issues and Care." www.apa.org/pi/eol/tasks.html

———. 2001b. "Issues of Access and Variability in Health Care at the End of Life." www.apa.org/pi/eol/access.html

———. 2003a. "Historical Changes Affecting End-of-Life Care." www.apa.org/pi/eol/historical.html

———. 2003b. "Terminology, Definitions, and Other Barriers to Communication." www.apa.org/pi/eol/terminology.html

———. 2003c. "Diversity Issues in End-of-Life Decision-Making." www.apa .org/pi/eol/diversity.html

———. 2003d. "Assisted Suicide." www.apa.org/pi/eol/arguments.html

———. 2004. "Mental Health Care and Older Adults." www.apa.org/ppo/ issues/oldermhfacto3.html

American Society on Aging. 1999. "Mentors Pass along Professional Legacy in Minority Aging." www.asaging.org/at/at-212/mentor_legacy.html

Amnesty International. 1998. "Prisoners Should Be Released Unconditionally on 15 August Freedom Anniversary." 13 August. www.amnestyusa.org/ news/1998/32052898.htm

Antieau, Kim. 2004. "Acting Locally." March 11. www.alternet.org/story/ 18099

Apologetics Index. 2001. "Americans' Belief in Psychic and Paranormal Phenomena Is Up Over Last Decade." www.apologeticsindex.org/news1/an010613-16 .html

Aristotle. 350 B.C.E. "On Youth and Old Age, On Life and Death, On Breathing." http://classics.mit.edu/Aristotle/youth_old.2.2.html

Armerding, Taylor. 2002. "Forget Smoking: Ageism Is the Real Threat." August 1. www.eagletribune.com/news/stories/20020801/LN_006.htm

Aronoff, C. 1974. "Old Age in Prime Time." *Journal of Communication* 24: 86–87.

Arthur, Chris. 2004. "A Revolution in Religious Consciousness." In *Religious Pluralism.* www.conexuspress.com/catalog/religious_pluralism_excerpt.htm

Asahi.com. 2004. "Planners Look to Old-timers to Rejuvenate Aging Society." http://news.shopeasier.com/files/shopeasier_Aging.htm

Asia, Inc. 1994. "Can Asia Afford Its Elderly?" December. www.saliltripathi .com/articlesAsiaInc/Dec94AsiaInc.html.

AskOxford. 2004. "World of Words." www.askoxford.com/worldofwords/ history/20thcentury/1930s/?view

Associated Press. 1998. "Dole Signs as Spokesman for Viagra." December 12. www .ljworld.com/section/article_about_bob_dole_story/139005

Association for Volunteer Administration. 2004. "Older Volunteers Enrich America Awards." www.avaintl.org/news/older_volunteer_award.html

Atchley, Robert C. 1995. "The Continuity of the Spiritual Self." In *Aging, Spirituality, and Religion,* ed. Melvin A. Kimble et al. Minneapolis: Fortress Press.

Atlantic Philanthropies. 2003. "About Atlantic." www.atlanticphilanthropies .org/about_atlantic/about_atlantic.asp

Austin, David, and Elizabeth M. Russell. 2003. "Is There Ageism in Oncology?" *Scottish Medical Journal* 48:17–20.

Awakening-Healing. 2004. "Healing from the Heart." www.awakening-healing .com/Healing.htm

Baicker, Katherine, and Amitabh Chandra. 2004. "Medicare Spending, Physician Workforce, and Beneficiaries' Quality of Care." *Health Affairs* 7 April, Datawatch W4-184.

Bass, Scott, Francis G. Caro, and Yung-Ping Chen, eds. 1993. *Achieving a Productive Society.* Westport, Conn.: Auburn House.

B.C. Indian Arts Society. 1982. *Martin Mungo.* Sidney, B.C.: Gray's Publishing.

Beard, George. 1881. *American Nervousness.* New York: G. P. Putnam's.

Beck, Ulrich. 1992. *Risk Society.* London: Sage Publishing.

Behrman, Greg. 2004. *The Invisible People: How the U.S. Has Slept through the Global AIDS Pandemic, the Greatest Humanitarian Catastrophe of Our Time.* New York: Free Press.

Bengtson, Vern L., and Ariela Lowenstein. 2003. *Global Aging and Challenges to Families.* New York: Aldine de Gruyter.

Bengtson, Vern L., Carolyn Rosenthal, and Linda Burton. 1995. "Paradoxes of Families and Aging." In *Handbook of Aging and the Social Sciences,* 4th ed., ed. Robert H. Binstock and Linda George, 253–82. San Diego: Academic Press.

Benson, Herbert. 1997. *Timeless Healing: The Power and Biology of Belief.* New York: Fireside.

Berkowitz, Edward D. 1991. *America's Welfare State from Roosevelt to Reagan.* Baltimore: Johns Hopkins University Press.

———. 2003. *Robert Ball and the Politics of Social Security.* Madison: University of Wisconsin Press.

Berman, Sanford. 1985. "Senior Citizens." *Unabashed Librarian* 56:17–19.

Bernstein, Carl. 1968. "Age and Race Fears Seen in Housing Opposition." *Washington Post,* March 7.

Berry, Thomas. 2001. "The Creative Role of Elders in the Human Community." *Second Journey* 1:1–7.

Bestler, Bob. 2004. "'Senior' Just Doesn't Cut It Anymore." www .myrtlebeachonline.com/mid/myrtlebeachonline/news/columnists/bob_ bestler/P

Bianchi, Eugene C. 1997. "Trans-traditional Spirituality." *Corpus Reports.* www .emory.edu/COLLEGE/RELIGION/faculty/bianchi/corpus97.htm

Biggs, Simon. 1999. *Mature Imagination.* Buckingham: Open University Press.

Binstock, Robert H. 2004. "Advocacy in an Era of Neo-Conservatism: Responses of National Aging Organizations." *Generations* 28:49–54.

Binstock, Robert H., and Jill Quadagno. 2001. "Aging and Politics." In *Handbook of Aging and the Social Sciences,* 5th ed., ed. Robert H. Binstock and Linda George. San Diego: Academic Press.

Birren, James E. 1955. "Speed of Response as a Function of Perceptual Difficulty and Age." *Journal of Gerontology* 10:429–36.

———, ed. 1996. *Encyclopedia of Gerontology,* 2 vols. San Diego: Academic Press.

Bishop, George. 1999. "What Americans Really Believe," *Free Inquiry Magazine* 19. www.secularhumanism.org/library/fi/bishop_19_3.html

Bleakney, Greg. 1994. "Initiation into the Heart of Life." www.menweb.org/ bleakney.htm

Blevins, Sue A. 1997. "Restoring Health Freedom," Cato Policy Analysis No. 290. www.cato.org/pubs/pas/[a-290.html

Bliss, Michael. 1999. *William Osler: A Life in Medicine.* Oxford: Oxford University Press.

Bluestone, Irving, Rhonda J. V. Montgomery, and John D. Owen, eds. 1990.

The Aging of the American Work Force. Detroit, Mich.: Wayne State University.

B'nai B'rith International. 2002. "Report." www.give.org

Bode, Carl. 1956. *The American Lyceum.* New York: Oxford University Press.

Bole, Kristen. 1997. "Adult Education Boom Gives College a Lesson in Business." *San Francisco Business Times.* http://sanfrancisco.bizjournals.com/sanfrancisco/stories/1997/02/04/focus3.html

Bork, Alfred. 2001. "Adult Education, Lifelong Learning, and the Future." www.ics.uci.edu/~bork/ADULTEDUCATION.htm

Bowling, Ann. 1999. "Ageism in Cardiology." *British Medical Journal* 319: 1353–55.

Bowman, Clive. 2001. "Governance and Autonomy in Alternatives to Hospital Care." *Age and Ageing* 30-S3:15–18.

Bradley, Dana Burr. 1999–2000. "A Reason to Rise Each Morning," *Generations* 45–49.

Breaux, John. 2003a. "Elderly Face Discrimination in Health Care, Experts Say." May 20. http://thedesertsun.com

———. 2003b. "Addressing Ageism in America's Healthcare System." July 11. www.senate.gov/~Breaux/columns/2003711356.html

Breen, Pam. 2003. "Not All Protestant Denominations Are Declining." PRWeb. www.prweb.com/releases/2003/11/prweb87640.php

British Geriatrics Society. 2001. "Influenza in Old Age." *Age and Ageing* 30: 361–63.

Bronte, Lydia. 1993. *The Longevity Factor.* New York: HarperCollins.

Brown, J. Douglas. 1977. *Essays on Social Security.* Princeton, N.J.: Princeton University, Industrial Relations Section.

Bruni, Frank. 2003. "Unraveling the Mortal Coil, in Plain View." *New York Times,* October 19, Sec. 4, p. 1.

Bukov, Aleksej, Ineke Maas, and Thomas Lampert. 2002. "Social Participation in the Very Old." *Journal of Gerontology: Psychological Sciences* 57B:P510–17.

Burns, Norman, and Cyril O. Houle, eds. 1948. *The Community Responsibilities of Institutions of Higher Learning.* Chicago: University of Chicago Press.

Bursztajn, Harold, and Archie Brodsky. 1999. "Captive Patients, Captive Doctors." *Forensic Psychiatry and Medicine.* www.forensic-psych.com

Bush, George W. 2002. Foreword. "Protecting the Civil Rights and Religious Liberty of Faith-Based Organizations." Washington, D.C.: White House Faith-Based and Community Initiatives.

Business Chronicle. 2000. "Companies Seeking Older Workers." www.augustachronicle.com/stories/060500/abc_companies.html

Business Women's Network. 2002. "Older Women." www.bwni.com

Butler, Robert N. 1975. *Why Survive? Being Old in America.* New York: Harper & Row.

———. 1998. "The Graying of Nations." International Longevity Center. www.ilcusa.org/who/senate/htm

———. 2003. "Ageism in Health Care." Testimony before U.S. Senate Special Committee on Aging. www.os.dhhs.gov/asl/testify/t030922.html

Butler, Robert N., Lawrence K. Grossman, and Mia R. Oberlink, eds. 1999. *Life in an Older America*. New York: Century Foundation Press.

Butler, Robert N., and Myrna J. Lewis. 1976. *Sex after Sixty*. New York: Harper & Row.

Butler, Stuart M. 2003. "Laying the Groundwork for Universal Health Care Coverage." Heritage Foundation. www.heritage.org/Research/HealthCare/testo31003.cfm

Byock, Ira R. 1998. "Hospice and Palliative Care." *Journal of Palliative Medicine* 1:165–76.

———. 1999. Testimony before U.S. House of Representatives Committee on Government Reform. www.dyingwell.com/uschrtest.htm

Byrd, Robert C. 2004. *Losing America*. New York: W. W. Norton.

Callahan, Daniel. 1987. *Setting Limits*. New York: Simon and Schuster.

———. 2003. *What Better Price Health?* Berkeley: University of California Press.

Callahan, Sidney. 2004. "A Feminist Case Against Self-Determined Dying in Assisted Suicide and Euthanasia." www.fnsa.org/vln4/callahan.html

Campbell, Andrea Louise, and Theda Skocpol. 2003. "Politics and the Elderly." www.yuricareport.com/Medicare/AARPsellsOutElderlyInMoreWays.html

Carlsen, Mary Baird. 1991. *Creative Aging*. New York: W. W. Norton.

Carmona, Richard H. 2003. "Testimony before Special Committee on Aging, U.S. Senate, Ageism in Healthcare." www.os.dhhs.gov/asl/testify/t030922.html

Carrese, Joseph A., Jamie L. Mullaney, Ruth R. Faden, and Thomas E. Finucane. 2002. "Planning for Death but Not Serious Future Illness." *British Journal of Medicine* 325:125–27.

Carson, Rachel. 1962. *Silent Spring*. Boston: Houghton Mifflin.

Carstensen, Laura, Barry Edelstein, and Laurie Dornbrand, eds. 1996. *The Practical Handbook of Clinical Gerontology*. Thousand Oaks, Calif.: Sage Publications.

Carter, Rosalynn. Institute for Caregiving. 2004. Brochure.

Catalog of Federal Domestic Assistance (CFDA). 2002. www.cfda.gov

Catholic Apologetics. 2004. "Euthanasia." www.geocities.com/cath_apolo/euthan.htm

Catholic Charities, Diocese of Pittsburgh. 2004. "Elderly Services." www.ccpgh.org/Website/elderly.htm

Catholic Charities USA. 2002. Report. www.give.org/reports/care_dyn.asp?109

CBSNews.com. 2004. "Doctors Guilty of Ageism." www.cbsnews.com/stories/2004/02/05/eveningnews/main598356.html

Center for Ageless Marketing. 2003. "Why Ageless Marketing?" www.agelessmarketing.com

Center for Democracy Studies. 1996. "The Promise Keepers Are Coming." highbeam.com/library/doco.asp?docid=161:187177032refid=ink_puballmegs

Center for Retirement Research. 2002. "Does the Social Security Earnings Test Affect Labor Supply and Benefits Receipt?" http://ideas/repec.org/p/crr/2000-07.html

Center for Social Gerontology. 1998. "Older Persons—Tobacco's Forgotten Victims." www.tcsg.org

Center for Spirituality and Healing, University of Minnesota. 2004. "About Us." www.csh.umn.edu/about/InTheNews/elder.html

Center for Strategic and International Studies (CSIS). 2004. "What Is the Global Aging Initiative?" www.csis.org/gai/

Center for Third Age Leadership. 2004. "Who Benefits from Third Age Planning?" www.thirdagecenter.com/benefits.htm

Center on an Aging Society. 2004. "Cultural Competence in Health Care." Issue Brief 5, Georgetown University.

CenterPoint. 2001. "For the Record." www.acenet.edu/calec/centerpoint/Issue_3/record/index.cfm

Centers for Disease Control and Prevention. 2003. "Life Expectancy at Birth." www.cdc.gov/nchs/data/us/tables/2003/03hus027.pdf

Chaleff, Ira. 2003. The Courageous Follower, 2d ed. New York: Berrett-Koehler.

Chapman, Julie. 2003. "Doctors Propose National Health Insurance." www.capitalnews9.com/content/health_team_9/?ArID=37233&SecID=17

Chapman, Steve. 2003. "Meet the Greedy Grandparents." December 10. http://slate.msn.com/id/2092302

Charrette. 2003. "Restoring a Sense of Place in Seattle's Nihonmachi." June 7. Draft document sponsored by Inter*Im Community Development Association.

Chavez, Linda. 1999. "Insight." Jewish World Review. www.jewishworldreview.com/cols/chavez033099.asp

Chinese Century. 2001. "Five-Year Plan Vows to Help Elderly." www.cnd.org/Global/01/08/26/010826-1.html

Chippendale, Lisa. 2004. "Spirituality, Religion and Healthy Aging." www.infoaging.org/feat9.html

Cho, David. 2002. "Evangelicals Help Lead U.S. Growth in Church Attendance during 1990s," Washington Post, September 17. www.-tech.mit.edu/V122/N40/long-5.40w.html

Ciba Foundation Symposium. 1988. Research and the Ageing Population. New York: John Wiley & Sons.

Cibuzar, Lynn. n.d. "From the Family Home to the Nursing Home: How to Ease Transition through Rituals." DARTS: Caregiver Support Services.

Clark, David Lee, ed. 1954. Shelley's Prose. Albuquerque: University of New Mexico Press.

Club of Rome. 1972. Limits to Growth. New York: Universe.

Cohen, Lizabeth. 1990. Making a New Deal. New York: Cambridge University Press.

Cole, Thomas R. 1992. The Journey of Life. New York: Cambridge University Press.

CommInfoStudies. 2004. "The Elderly and the Media." www.uky.edu/CommInfoStudies/JAT/Telecommunications/Faculty_Staff/Jim.html

Committee on the Present Danger. 2004. "This Generation's War Must Be Won." New York Times, July 21.

Community Without Walls. 2003. "A Pilot Study for Widening Horizons." www.princetonol.com/groups/cww

Compassion in Dying. 2004. www.compassionindying.org/

Conway, Christopher. 1998. *Strategies for Mentoring.* New York: John Wiley & Sons.

Conwell, Yeates. 2002. "Older White Men a High Suicide Risk." www.msnbc.com/avantgo/774719.htm

Council of Europe. 2000. "Improving the Status and Role of Volunteers as a Contribution by the Parliamentary Assembly to the International Year of Volunteers 2001." http://assembly.coe.int/Documents/WorkingDocs/Doc00/EDOC8917.htm

Courier-Journal.com. 2004. "Empty Pulpits." April 4. www.courier-journal.com/cjextra/2004projects/empty_pulpits/day1/A1-pastors0404-1

Cowdry, Edmund Vincent, ed. 1939. *Problems of Ageing.* Baltimore: Williams and Wilkins.

———. 1941. *Problems of Ageing,* 2d ed. Baltimore: Williams and Wilkins.

Cox, Harvey. 1968. "The Secular Search for Religious Experience." www.theologytoday.ptsem.edu/oct1968/v25-3-article4.htm

Craemer, Mary Lou. 2003. "Mainline Churches Again Filling Pews." May 25. www.thetimesherald.com/news/stories/20030525/localnews/365206.html

Crane, David. 2004. "Aging Society a Threat and an Opportunity." www.lawrencehartman.com_news_stvd/01_05_04.htm

Cremin, Lawrence. 1970–88. *American Education.* 3 vols. New York: Harper Torchbooks.

Csikszentmihalyi, Mihaly. 1995. "Creativity Across the Life Span: A Systems View." *Davidson Institute for Talent Development.* http://print.ditd.org/floater=171.html

Cutler, Neal, Nancy Whitelaw, and Bonita L. Beattie. 2002. *American Perceptions of Aging in the Twenty-first Century.* Washington, D.C.: National Council on the Aging.

Cutter, John A. 2003. "Spirituality May Help People Live Longer." www.klinikong.com/spiritual/

Dagastino, Paul. 1997. "Senior Citizens Vote 'No' on Schools, but Volunteer." *Business Journal.* www.bizjournals.com/phoenix/stories/1997/08/11/focus9.html.

Dahlberg, Steven. 2004. "The New Elderhood," February. (PDF) http://agescan.blogspot.com

Dallach, Marie. 1933. "Old Age, American Style." *New Outlook* 162:50.

Daniels, Norman. 1988. *Am I My Parents' Keeper?* New York: Oxford University Press.

Dartmouth Medical School, Center for Evaluative Clinical Sciences. 1998. *The Dartmouth Atlas of Health Care, 1998.* American Hospital Publishing Co.

Davis, Karen. 2004. "Making Health Care Affordable for All Americans." Testimony before the Senate Committee on Health, Education, Labor, and Pensions. January 28.

Davis, Kenneth G. 1994. *Primero Dios: Alcoholics Anonymous and the Hispanic Community.* Selinsgrove, Pa.: Susquehanna University Press.

Day, Christine. 1990. *What Older Americans Think*. Princeton, N.J.: Princeton University Press.

Deets, Horace B. 2001. "Build Bridges to Elders, Not Generational Fences," *Aging Today*. www.asaging.org/at/at-219/Forum.html

DeLagun, Frederica. 1963. "Mungo Martin." *American Anthropologist* 65: 894–96.

deLeon, Ferdinand M. 1999. "Revisiting the Life and Legacy of Pioneering Filipino Writer Carlos Bulosan." August 8. www.reflectionsofasia.com/carlosbulosan.htm

Della Santina, Peter. 1989. "Buddhism in Practice." ww.ecst.csuchico.edu/~dsantina/prac3.htm

Delloff, Linda-Marie. 1987. "Distorted Images: The Elderly and the Media." *Christian Century*, January 7–14.

Del Monte Foods. 2001. "Del Monte Foods to Receive Governor's Exemplary Employer Award." Press release. www.delmonte.com/Company/release/press33.htm

Denneen, Bill. 2000. "Eye of the Storm." www.overpopulation.org/forum.html

Derr, Erik. 2002. "Uncle Bob's Chinatown." April 4–10. www.asianweek.com/2002_04_05/news_unclebob.html

Dewey, John. 1937. *Reconstruction in Philosophy*. Boston: Beacon Press.

———. 1939. "Introduction." In *Problems of Ageing,* ed. Edmund V. Cowdry. Baltimore: Williams and Wilkins.

Dionne, E. J., Jr., and Ming Hsu Chen. 2001. *Sacred Places, Civic Purposes*. Washington, D.C.: Brookings Institution.

Divorce Magazine. 2003. www.divorcemag.com/statistics/statsUS.shtml

Divorce Reform. 2003. www.divorcereform.org.rates.html

Dixon, Om. 2004. AIDS. www.thirdage.com/features/healthy/aids/

Dodd, Nigel. 1999. *Social Theory and Modernity*. London: Polity Press.

Dorgan, Charity Ann. 1996. *Statistical Record of Older Americans*, 2d ed. Detroit: Gale Publishing.

Dorland, W. A. Newland. 1908. *The Age of Mental Virility*. New York: Century Co.

Dowell, John A. 1998. "To Be a Citizen." www.msu.edu/user/vandrag2/ATL135/Citizen.htm

Dower, John A. 1999. *Embracing Defeat*. New York: W. W. Norton.

Duke University. 1999. "Religious Attendance Linked to Lower Mortality in the Elderly." News Release.

Dunn, William. 1992. *Selling the Story*. Ithaca, N.Y.: American Demographics Books.

Dychtwald, Ken. 2003a. "The Age Wave Is Coming." *PM Magazine*. www.icma.org/pm/8506/Dychtwald.htm

———. 2003b. "How the Coming Longevity Revolution Will Transform the Marketplace, the Workplace and Our Lives." www.agewave.com/media_files/longevity.html

Economic Council. 1983. *Japan in the Year 2000*. Tokyo: Japan Times, Ltd.

Egemin Worldwide. 2004. "Wanted: Twenty Years Experience." www.egemin.com/country/template.html?id=209

Ekerdt, David J. 2004a. "Born to Retire: The Foreshortened Life Course." *The Gerontologist* 44:3–9.

———. 2004b. "Consumption and Meanings of Age." *Journal of Gerontology: Social Sciences* 59B:S57.

Elderhostel. 2004. "What Is Elderhostel?" www.elderhostel.org/about/what_is.asp

Elders Camp. 2004. "Elders Leadership Training Camp-Basic Concept." www.arcticoutreach.org/elderscamp.html

Eliot, T. S. 1952. *The Complete Poems and Plays.* New York: Harcourt, Brace, and World.

Ellis, James B., Amy S. Bruckman, and Richard Satterwhite. n.d. "Children and Elders Sharing Stories: Lessons from Two Online Oral History Projects." Contact: jellis@cc.gatech.edu

Ellison, Christopher G. 1998. "Religion, Health, and Well-Being among African-Americans." www.rcgd.isr/umich/edu/prba/perspectives/spring1998/cellison2/pdf

End-of-Life Choices. 2004. Website. www.hemlock.org/index.jsp

Enfield, Susan, and Linda Formichelli. 2005. "Lessons from Grandma." www.allaboutaging.com/allaboutaging/lessons.html

English, Jane. 1993. "What Do Grown Children Owe Their Parents?" In *Vice and Virtue in Everyday Life,* ed. C. Sommers and F. Sommers, 758–65. Ft. Worth, Tex.: Harcourt.

Environmental League. 2002. "The Massachusetts Environment: Selected Issues for the 2002 Campaign." www.environmentalleague.org/issues_paper.html

Episcopal Senior Ministries. 2002. "A Study of Three, Diverse, Minority Senior Populations in the Episcopal Diocese of Washington, D.C."

———. 2004. "About Us." www.esm.org/about.htm

Eric Digests. 1991. "Older Worker Training." www.ericdigests.org/pre-9220/older.htm

———. 1995. "Older Workers in Transition." listserv.ed.gov/archives/edinfo/archived/msg00261.html

Espinosa, Gaston, Virgilio Elizondo, and Jesse Miranda. 2003. "Hispanic Churches in American Public Life." Interim Reports. Institute for Latino Studies, University of Notre Dame.

Estes, Richard J. 2004. PRAXIS. Caster.ssw.upenn.edu/~restes/praxis.html

European Social Welfare Information Network. 1999. "International: Population Groups: Elderly." www.eswin.net/int/eld.htm

Fagan, Patrick F. 1996. "Why Religion Matters." *The Heritage Foundation.* January 25. www.heritage.org/Research/Religion/BG1064.cfm

Fairgrove, Rowan. 2004. "Links to Multifaith and Religion Sites." www.conjure.com/religion.htm

Fallot, Roger D. 1998. *Spirituality and Religion in Recovery from Mental Illness.* San Francisco: Jossey-Bass Publishers.

Fass, Paula. 1978. *The Damned and the Beautiful.* New York: Oxford University Press.

Fays, Edward. 2002. *A Grandparent's Gift of Love.* New York: Warner Books.

Featherstone, Mike. 1991. *Consumer Culture and Postmodernism*. London: Sage.

———. 1995. *Undoing Culture: Globalization, Postmodernism, and Identity*. London: Sage.

Fischer, David Hackett. 1977. *Growing Old in America,* expanded edition. New York: Oxford University Press.

Fischer, Kathleen. 1998. *Winter Grace*. Nashville: Upper Room Books.

Fischer, Lucy Rose, and Kay Bannister Schaffer. 2004. "The Future of Old Age." *Energize*. www.energizeinc.com/art/aold.html

Fisher, Deborah. 2003. *Assets in Action*. Minneapolis: Search Institute.

Flexner, Stuart Berg. 1982. *Listening to America*. New York: Simon and Schuster.

Foner, Eric, and John A. Garraty, eds. 1991. *The Reader's Companion to American History*. Boston: Houghton Mifflin.

Forman, Maurice Buxton, ed. 1952. *The Letters of John Keats*. Oxford: Oxford University Press.

Fox, Richard Wightman, and T. J. Jackson Lears, ed. 1983. *The Culture of Consumption*. New York: Pantheon.

Francher, J. 1973. "It's the Pepsi Generation." *International Journal of Aging and Human Development* 4:245–55.

Franz, Leslie. 1999. "Mental Illness and the Elderly." *UCSD Health Sciences*. www.ucsdnews.ucsd.edu

Freedman, David Noel, ed. 1992. *The Anchor Bible Dictionary,* 6 vols. New York: Doubleday.

Freedman, Marc. 1993. *The Kindness of Strangers*. San Francisco: Jossey-Bass.

———. 1999. *Prime Time*. New York: Public Affairs.

Friedan, Betty. 1993. *The Fountain of Age*. New York: Simon and Schuster.

Friedland, Robert B., and Laura Summer. 1999. *Demography Is Not Destiny*. Washington, D.C.: National Academy for an Aging Society.

Friedman, Valerie. 2004. "The Hemlock Society." http://members.aol.com/fcisct/Hemlock_Society.htm

Frogue, James. 2001. *Top Ten Ways to Fix America's Health Insurance and Expand Coverage*. Washington, D.C.: The Heritage Foundation.

Fronstin, Paul. 2004. "The Impact on Employment-Based Health Benefits of the Shift from a Manufacturing Economy to a Service Economy." *Employee Benefit Research Institute* 25:1–7.

Fuchs, Mark. 2003. "New Clerics Seek Ways to Reach Aging Flocks." *New York Times,* August 9, A11.

Gafni, Marc. 2003. *The Mystery of Love*. New York: ATRIA Books.

Galenson, David W. 2003. The Two Life Cycles of Human Creativity. *NEBR Reporter: Research Summary*. www.nber.org/reporter/fa1103/galenson.html

Garbl's Writing Center. 2004. "Style Manual: E;" "Style Manual: S." http://garbl.home.comcast.net/stylemanual/e.htm

Gearon, Christopher J. 2003. "A Matter of Life and Death." December. www.aarp.org/bulletin/yourhealth/Articles/a2003-12-09-livingwill.html

Geipel, Gary L. 2003. "Global Aging and the Global Workforce." http://wd.hudson.org/index.cfm?fuseaction=publication_details&id=2740

Generations. 1996. "Legacies." American Society on Aging publication no. 20.

Generations United. 2004a. "Intergenerational Program Database." www.gu
.org/prog.htm
———. 2004b. "Fact Sheet." Washington, D.C.
Gergen, Kenneth J., and Mary M. Gergen. 2004. "The New Aging." www.trinity
.edu/~mkearl/geropsy.html
Gerontological Society of America. 2003. "Online Resources in Aging." www
.geron.org/online.html
Geteducated.com. 2004. "Distance Learning Consulting, Research and News."
www.geteducated.com
Getzen, Thomas E. 1992. "Population Aging and the Growth of Health Expen-
ditures." *Journal of Gerontology: Social Sciences* 47:S98–104.
Giddens, Anthony. 1990. *The Consequences of Modernity.* Stanford, Calif.:
Stanford University Press.
Gilleard, Chris, and Paul Higgs. 2000. *Cultures of Ageing.* New York: Prentice-
Hall.
Gillick, Muriel R. 1994. *Choosing Medical Care in Old Age.* Cambridge, Mass.:
Harvard University Press.
Gilmore, Janet. 2002. "Youths More Conservative Than Their Elders on Issues
Involving Religion and Abortion, New UC Berkeley Survey Reveals." *Cam-
pus News.* www.berkeley.edu/news/media/releases/2002/09/24_youth.html
Global Action on Aging. 2004. "Elder Rights: World." http://globalag.igc.org/
elderrights/world/
Goldberg, Beverly. 2000. *Age Works.* New York: Free Press.
Gondolf, Edward W. 1999. "Alcohol Treatment for the Older Patient." *Mid-
Atlantic Addiction Training Institute.* Indiana University of Pennsylvania.
Goodenough, Patrick. 2003. "Hemlock Society Disavows Radical's Views." Jan-
uary 17. www.cnsnews.com/ForeignBureau/Archive/200302/FOR20030117a
.html
Graebner, William. 1980. *A History of Retirement.* New Haven, Conn.: Yale
University Press.
Grandparents for Children's Rights. 2004. www.grandparentsforchildren.org/
menu.htm
Grant, Lynda D. 1996. "The Effects of Ageism on Individual and Health Care
Providers' Responses to Healthy Aging." *Health and Social Work* 21:9–15.
Grantmakers in Aging. 2004. "What's New on the GIA Website." www.giaging
.org
Greenspan, Alan. 2003. "Aging Global Population." Testimony before the U.S.
Senate, Special Committee on Aging. www.federalreserve.gov/boarddocs/
testimony/2003/20030227
Greenstein, Robert. 2000. "The Earnings Test and Social Security." www/cbpp
.org/2-15-00socsec.htm
Griffin, David Ray. 1988. *Spirituality and Society.* Albany: State University of
New York Press.
Griffith, Robert W. 2002. "Looking after Grandmother." *Health and Age.*
www.healthandage.com
Griswold, Frank T. 2004. "Humanitarian Crisis Remains Unaddressed." *The
Living Church,* July 25, 9.

Groopman, Jerome. 2004. *The Anatomy of Hope*. New York: Random House.

Gruman, Gerald J. 1966. (2003). *A History of Ideas about the Prolongation of Life*. New York: Springer Publishing.

Gullette, Margaret Morganroth. 2004. *Aged by Culture*. Chicago: University of Chicago Press.

Haber, Carole. 1983. *Beyond Sixty-Five*. New York: Cambridge University Press.

Haber, Carole, and Brian Gratton. 1994. *Old Age and the Search for Security*. Bloomington: Indiana University Press.

Haddad, Yvonne Yazbeck. 1991. *The Muslims of America*. New York: Oxford University Press.

Hagelberg, Kymberli. 1997. "Death: Is It a Dying Patient's Last Right?" March 20. www.sunnews.com

Hall, G. Stanley. 1904. *Adolescence*. New York: D. Appelton & Sons.

———. 1922. *Senescence*. New York: D. Appelton & Sons.

Hall, Melissa. 2003. "Companies Seeking Older Workers." *Business Chronicle*. www.augustachronicle.com/stories/060500/abc_companies.shtml

Haller, D. J. 1998. "Alcoholics Anonymous and Spirituality." *Social Work and Christianity* 25:101–14.

Hall of Fame. 2003. "Beverly Benner Cassara." www.occe.ou.edu/hallofame/2003/Cassara.html

Harris, Corra. 1926. "The Borrowed Timers." *Ladies Home Journal* 43:35.

Harris, Diana K. 1988. *Dictionary of Gerontology*. Westport, Conn.: Greenwood Press.

Hart, Mary. 2001. "There Is a Silver Lining to Global Aging." May 23. www.post-gazette.com/neigh_south/20010523smaryhart9.asp

Haskell, Kari. 2004. "Older Volunteers Give Back, and Find They Get Back, Too." *New York Times,* January 25, p. 23.

Hastings Center. 1987. *Guidelines on the Termination of Life-Sustaining Treatment and the Care of the Dying*. Bloomington: Indiana University Press.

Hauprich, Ann. 2004. "Men Combine Works, Prayer." www.evangelist.org/archive/hm/0724mens.htm

Hauser, Philip M., and Raul Vargas. 1960. "Population Structure and Trends." In *Aging in Western Societies,* ed. Ernest Burgess. Chicago: University of Chicago Press.

Hawksworth, John. 2002. "Seven Key Effects of Global Aging." www.pwcglobal.com/

Hawthorn, Audrey. 1979. *Kwakiutl Art*. Seattle: University of Washington Press.

Hayflick, Leonard. 1994. *How and Why We Age*. New York: Ballantine Books.

HCR Manor Care. 2002–2003. "Grant List." www.hcr-manorcare.org

Health and Age. 2004. "Does Ageism Affect Health Care Rationing?" *Health and Age.com*. www.healthandage.com/html/res/healthpolicy/content.page3.htm

HealthCentral. 2001. "Elderly Rarely Die of 'Old Age.'" www.junkscience.com/Sep01.htm

Health-Minder. 1999. "Ageism: Medical Aspects." www.health-minder.com/HealthMinderNews/Nov99

Health Resources and Services Administration. 2004. *A National Agenda for Geriatric Education.* www.bhpr.hrsa.gov/interdisciplinary/gecrec/gecrecallhlth.html

Healthy Senior. 2002. "Global Aging Threatens World's Economies." www.applesforhealth.com/HealthySenior/gloathwe3.html

Held, David. 1999. *Global Transformation.* Stanford: Stanford University Press.

Hendershot, Gerry. 2002a. "People Seeking Pastoral Care More Likely to Have Disability." www.nod.org/content.cfm?id=874

———. 2002b. "People with Disabilities Are More Likely to Pray for Health." www.nod/org/content.cfm?id=1475

Hendricks, Jon, Laurie Russell Hatch, and Stephen J. Cutler. 1999. "Entitlements, Social Compacts, and the Trend toward Retrenchment in U.S. Old-Age Programs." *Hallym International Journal of Aging* 1:14–31.

Hiemstra, Roger. 1993. "Older Women's Ways of Learning." http://home.twcny.rr.com/hiemstra/unospeech.html

Higgins, Mark. 1994. "Reflections of Seattle's Chinese Americans." August 29. http://seattlepi.nwsource.com/neighbors/id/reflect19.html

———. 1996. "A Place Asian Elders Can Call Home." http://seattlepi.nwsource.com/neighbors/id/vil119.html

———. 1997. "What Should You Call Seattle's Asian Neighborhood? Here's One Solution." June 7. http://seattlepi.nwsource.com/neighbors/id/name19.html

———. 2004. "Old Associations Hold Little Appeal for New Generations" http://seattlepi.nwsource.com/neighbors/id/assn19.html

Hippocrates. *Hippocrates,* vol. 1. Trans. W. H. S. Jones. Cambridge, Mass.: Harvard University Press, 1948.

HistoryLink.org. 2004. "Seattle Neighborhoods." www.historylink.org/output.cfm?file_id=1058

Hitchcock, John. 1991. *The Web of the Universe: Jung, the "New Physics" and Human Spirituality.* New York: Paulist Press.

Hobbs, Frank B., and Bonnie L. Damon. 1996. *65+ in the United States.* Washington, D.C.: U.S. Bureau of the Census. Current Population Reports, Special Studies, P23–190.

Hodkinson, H. D. 1975. *An Outline of Geriatrics.* London: Academic Press.

Holtz, Debra Levi. 2003. "Serving Elders Becomes Calling for Reutlinger's Spiritual Leader." www.jewishsf.com/bk030711/suppo3.shtml

Holtzman, Abraham. 1975. *The Townsend Movement.* New York: Octagon Books.

hooks, bell. 1994. *Teaching to Transgress.* New York: Routledge.

Hornblower, Simon, and Antony Spawforth, eds. 1996. *The Oxford Classical Dictionary,* 3d ed. Oxford: Oxford University Press.

Hudson, Robert. 1978. "The 'Graying' of the Federal Budget and Its Consequences for Old Age Policy." *The Gerontologist* 18:428–40.

Ibe, Hideo. 2000. *Aging in Japan.* New York: International Longevity Center.

Ignatieff, Michael. 2004. *The Lesser Evil.* Princeton, N.J.: Princeton University Press.

Infed. 2004. "Eduard Lindeman and Informal Education." www.infed.org/thinkers/et-lind.htm

Institute for Research on Women and Gender. 2002. "Aging in the Twenty-first Century." Consensus Report. Stanford University.

Institute of Medicine. 1999. "Ensuring Quality Cancer Care." www.nap.edu/books/0309064805/html

Interfaith Ministries. 2004. "IVC Mission Statement." www.chron.com/content/community/religious

Inter*Im. 2002. "History." www.interimicda.org/history.shtml

International Association of Gerontology. 2003. *Research Agenda on Ageing for the Twenty-first Century.* With the United Nations Programme on Ageing. Vancouver: Simon Fraser University.

International District. 2001. "Celebrating the Diverse Cultures of Asia." www.internationaldistrict.org/history.asp

———. 2004. Fact Index. www.fact-index.com/i/international_district_seattle_washington.html

International Federation on Ageing. 2004. Homepage. www.ifa-fiv.org

International Longevity Center. 2004. Homepage. www.ilcusa.org

International Religious Foundation. 1995. *World Scripture.* St. Paul, Minn.: Paragon House.

Intrados USA. 2003. "Findings from a New National Survey of Older Americans about Their Current and Future Needs." www.intrados.org/findings_from_national_sur.htm

Irwin, Lee. 2004. "Western Esotericism, Eastern Spirituality, and the Global Future." www.esoteric.msu.edu/Volume III/HTML/Irwin.html

Ives, Nat. 2004. "Advertising." *New York Times,* January 12, C8.

Jackson, William A. 1998. *The Political Economy of Population Ageing.* Cheltenham, UK: Edward Elgar.

Jacobs, Jane. 1961. *The Death and Life of Great American Cities.* New York: Random House.

———. 2004. *Dark Age Ahead.* New York: Random House.

JAHF (John A. Hartford Foundation). 2005. Homepage. www.jhartfound.org

James, Gregory. 2004. "Addressing Barriers to Health Care for Our Elderly." American College of Osteopathic Family Physicians.

James, William. 1890. *Principles of Psychology,* 2 vols. New York: Henry Holt.

———. 1901–2. *The Varieties of Religious Experience.* New York: Modern Library [1936].

Jennings, M. Kent, and Hazel Markus. 1988. "Political Involvement in Later Years." *American Journal of Political Science* 32:302–16.

Jewell, Albert, ed. 1999. *Spirituality and Ageing.* London: Jessica Kingsley.

Jewish Home and Hospital Lifecare System. 2004. "About Us." www.jewishhome.org

Jobe, Hazel. 1999. "Senior Pals: Bridging the Generation Gap with Technology." *Education World.* www.education-world.com/a_curr/curr159.shtml

John, Robert. 2004. "American Indian Elderly." http://socrates.berkeley.edu/aging/ModuleMinority1.html

Johns Hopkins Health System. 1999. "Celebrating the Contributions of William Osler." www.medicalarchives.jhmi.edu/osler/osler

Johnson, Donald E. L. 2002. "U.S. Needs Community Rates for Health Risks." *Health Strategic Management* 20:1–3.

Johnson, Harold R. 1995. "Claiming Boundaries." *Generations* 19:23–24.

Johnson, Paul. 1987. "The Structured Dependency of the Elderly: A Critical Note." London: Centre for Economic Policy Research.

Jonaitis, Aldona, ed. 1991. *The Enduring Kwakiutl Potlatch*. Seattle: University of Washington Press.

Jossey-Bass. 2004. "New Directions for Adult and Continuing Education: Complete List of Issues." www.josseybass.com/WileyCDA/Section/id-5507.html

Journal of Extension. 1992. "Older Volunteers Leading the Way." www.joe.org/joe/1992fall/a1.html

Julian, Norman. 2001. "Spirituality, Religion Play a Part in the Healing Process." www.dominionpost.com/a/news/2001/05/07/ba/

Jurek, John. 1996. "Why I'm Dancing Now." www.menweb.org/jurek.htm

Kahn, Joseph. 2004. "The Most Populous Nation Faces a Population Crisis." *New York Times,* May 30, "Week in Review."

Kaiser, Frank. 2004. "I Say Senior, You Say Señor." www.suddenlysenior.com/boomerhatesenior.html

Kane, Robert L., David H. Solomon, John C. Beck, Emmett B. Keeler, and Rosalie A. Kane. 1981. *Geriatrics in the United States*. Lexington, Mass.: Lexington Books.

Kateb, George. 1963. *Utopia and Its Enemies*. Glencoe: Free Press.

Katz, Jay. 2002. *The Silent World of Doctor and Patient*. Baltimore: Johns Hopkins University Press.

Katz, Stephen. 1999. "Old Age as Lifestyle in an Active Society." *Occasional Papers of the Doreen B. Townsend Center for the Humanities,* no. 19. University of California, Berkeley.

Katz, Stephen, and Barbara Marshall. 2003. "New Sex for Old: Lifestyle, Consumerism, and the Ethics of Aging Well." *Journal of Aging Studies* 17:3–16.

Kaveny, M. Cathleen. 1998. "Older Women and Health Care." *America*. www.americamagazine.org/articles/KavenyOlder.htm

Keegan, Desmond, ed. 1993. *Theoretical Principles of Distance Education*. London: Routledge.

Kelly, Tom. 2003. "Stereotypes Avoided When 'Function' Emphasized over 'Age'." http://www.inman.com/cb/story.asp?ID=38610

Kent, Heather. 1999. "Breast Cancer Treatment and Older Women." *Canadian Medical Journal Association* 161:15.

Kerka, Sandra. 1999. "Creativity in Adulthood." *Eric Digests*. www.ericdigests.org/1999-4/creativity.htm

Kertzer, David I., and Peter Laslett, eds. 1994. *Aging in the Past: Demography, Society, and Old Age*. Berkeley: University of California Press.

Kett, Joseph. 1977. *Rites of Passage*. New York: Basic Books.

———. 1994. *The Pursuit of Knowledge Under Difficulties*. Stanford, Calif.: Stanford University Press.

Kettl, Donald F. 2000. *The Global Public Management Revolution*. Washington, D.C.: Brookings Institution.

Keyser, Cheryl H. 2003. "The Importance of Civic Engagement to Older Americans." *Innovations,* Issue 2, National Council on the Aging, 9–14.

Kieffer, Jerold A. 1986. "The Older Volunteer Reserve." www.nap.edu

Kim, Jungmeen E., and Phyllis Moen. 2002. "Retirement Transitions, Gender, and Psychological Well-being: A Life-course, Ecological Model." *Journal of Gerontology: Psychological Sciences* 57B:P212–22.

Kimble, Mel, Susan H. McFadden, James Ellor, and James J. Seeber, eds. 1995. *Aging, Spirituality, and Religion.* Minneapolis: Fortress Press.

King's Fund. 2000. *Briefing Note: Age Discrimination in Health and Social Care.* London: King's Fund.

Kirby, Sarah E., Peter G. Coleman, and Dave Daley. 2004. "Spirituality and Well-Being in Frail and Nonfrail Older Adults." *Journal of Gerontology: Psychological Sciences* 59B: P123–29.

Kleinfield, N. R. 2004a. "In Death Watch for a Stranger, Becoming a Friend to the End." *New York Times,* January 25.

———. 2004b. "Old Patients, Hoping to Make Doctors Better." *New York Times,* June 17, A25.

Knowles, Malcolm S., Elwood F. Holton III, and Richard A. Swanson. 1998. *The Adult Learner,* 5th ed. Houston, Tex.: Gulf Publishing Company.

Koch, Adrienne, and William Peden, eds. 1944. *The Life and Selected Writings of Thomas Jefferson.* New York: Modern Library.

Koenig, Harold G. 1994. *Aging and God: Spiritual Pathways to Mental Health in Midlife and Later Years.* New York: Haworth Press.

———. 1995. "Religion and Health in Later Years." In *Aging, Spirituality, and Religion,* ed. Melvin A. Kimble et al. Minneapolis: Fortress Press.

———. 1999. *The Healing Power of Faith: Science Explores Medicine's Last Great Frontier.* New York: Simon and Schuster.

Koenig, Harold G., and Harvey Jay Cohen, eds. 2002. *The Link between Religion and Health: Psychoneuroimmunology and the Faith Factor.* New York: Oxford University Press.

Koenig, Harold G., and Douglas M. Lawson. 2004. *Faith in the Future: Healthcare, Aging, and the Role of Religion.* Philadelphia: Templeton Foundation Press.

Kokkola, Sari. 1998. "Why Don't We Always Call a Spade a Spade?" www.uta.fi/FAST/US1/Pl/SLA/skspade.html

Konrad, Rachel. 2001. "Tech Ageism Works Both Ways." www.globalaging.org/elderrights/US/tech.htm

Kosmin, Barry A., Egon Mayer, and Ariela Keysar. 2001. *American Religious Identification Survey, 2001.* New York: Graduate Center of the City of New York.

Krauss, Clifford. 2004. "War? Terrorists? No, Here's What's Really Scary." *New York Times,* June 29, C18.

Kubler, George. 1962. *The Shape of Time.* New Haven, Conn.: Yale University Press.

Kumashiro, Masaharu, ed. 2003. *Aging and Work.* London: Taylor & Francis.

Kurtz, Ernest. 1979. *Not-God: A History of Alcoholics Anonymous.* Center City, Minn.: Hazelden Educational Services.

Lamdin, Lois, with Mary Fulgate. 1997. *Elderlearning*. Washington, D.C.: American Council on Education.

Lansing, Albert I., ed. 1952. *Cowdry's Problems of Ageing*, 3d ed. Baltimore: Williams & Wilkins.

Larson, David B. 1993. *The Faith Factor: Volume Two*. Bethesda: National Institute for Healthcare Research.

Last Acts Partnership. 2004. www.partnershipforcaring.org/HomePage/content .html

Lawrence, Steven. 2002. "Children and Youth Funding Update." Foundation Center. http://fdncenter.org

League of Women Voters. 2003. "A Prescription for Universal, Affordable Health Care." www.globalaging.org/elderrights/us/lwv.htm

Learned, William S. 1924. *The American Public Library and the Diffusion of Knowledge*. New York: Harcourt, Brace.

Learnframe. 2001. "about e-learning." www.learnframe.com/aboutelearning/ page19.asp

Lebowitz, Barry. 2004. "Clinical Trials in Late Life: New Science in Old Paradigms." *The Gerontologist* 44:452–58.

Leech, Kenneth. 1992. *The Eye of the Storm*. New York: HarperCollins.

Leege, David C., and Thomas A. Trozzolo. n.d. *Report no. 3: Participation in Catholic Parish Life: Religious Rites and Parish Activities in the 1980s*. University of Notre Dame: Notre Dame Study of Catholic Parish Life.

Lehman, Harvey C. 1953. *Aging and Achievement*. Princeton, N.J.: Princeton University Press.

Lehrman, Leonard. 2002. "Reflections on the Shoah and Refuge Down Under." http://ljlehrman.artists-in-residence.com

Levin, Jeffrey S., ed. 1994. *Religion in Aging and Health: Theoretical Foundations and Methodological Frontiers*. Thousand Oaks, Calif.: Sage Publications.

———. 2001. *God, Faith, and Health: Exploring the Spirituality-Healing Connection*. New York: John Wiley & Sons.

Levine, Wayne M. 2001. "Men, Psychology and Spirituality in a Shame-Based Society." www.westcoastmenscenter.com/article1.htm

Lewis, Laurie. 2002. "Intergenerational Programs That Really Work." www .amda.com/caring/august2002/intergenerational.htm

Liang, Jersey, Joan Bennett, Neal Krause, Erika Kobayashi, Hyekyung Kim, J. Winchester Brown, Hiroko Akiyama, Hidehiro Sugiwasa, and Arvind Jain. 2002. "Old Age Mortality in Japan." *Journals of Gerontology* 57B: S294–307.

Lindeman, Eduard C. 1926. *The Meaning of Adult Education*. New York: New Republic.

Lipson, Lois. 1994. "Senior Citizens as School Volunteers." *Eric Digests*. www .ericdigests.1994/senior/htm

Living Church. 2003. "Alternative Court for Disputes between Christians." November 16.

Loeb, Paul Rogat. 1999. *Soul of a Citizen*. New York: St. Martin's Griffin.

Longman, Phillip. 1987. *Born to Pay*. Boston: Houghton Mifflin Co.

Lorenz, Kate. 2005, February 16. "Say Goodbye to Traditional Retirement." http://findajob.aol.com/findajob/articles/article.adp?id=602

Lumpkin, James, Marjorie J. Cabellero, and Lawrence B. Chonko. 1989. *Direct Marketing, Direct Selling, and the Mature Consumer.* New York: Quorum Books.

MacIntosh, Heather. 2003. "How Affordable Housing Incentive Programs Fund Preservation." www.cityofseattle.net/commnty/histsea/preservationseattle/publicpolicy/defaultjune

MacIntyre, Alasdair. 1981. *After Virtue.* Notre Dame, Ind.: Notre Dame University Press.

Mackinnon, Neil J., Jeffrey D. Molson, and J. Douglas May. 2003. "Physician Interventions in the Dying Process." *Electronic Journal of Sociology.* www.sociology.org/content/vo17.1/mackinnon_etal.html

Maddox, George L., ed. 1995. *Encyclopedia of Aging,* 2d ed. New York: Springer Publishing.

Malley, Paul. 2004. "The Clergy's Journal." February. www.agingwithdignity.org/clergy.html

Manheimer, Ronald, ed. 1994. *Older Americans Almanac.* Detroit: Gale Publishing.

Marshall, Barbara, and Stephen Katz. 2002. "Forever Functional: Sexual Fitness and the Ageing Male Body." *Body and Society* 8:43–70.

Marshall, Tom. 2000. "Ageism Occurs in Prevention of Heart Disease Too." *British Medical Journal* 320:1077.

Martin, James Kirby, Randy Roberts, Steven Mintz, Linda O. McMurry, and James H. Jones. 2000. *America and Its Peoples,* 4th ed. New York: Longman.

Martin, Lillien J. 1944. *A Handbook for Old Age Counselors.* San Francisco: Geertz Printing Co.

Martin, Lillien J., and Clare DeGruchy. 1930. *Salvaging Old Age.* New York: Macmillan.

May, Timothy D. 2001. "Dedicated Senior Citizens Keep Watch over Pennsylvania Waterways." www.citizenreviewonline.org/Dec_2001/volunteers_monitor.htm

McClure, Charles R., and John Carlo Bertot. 1998. *Public Library Use in Pennsylvania: Identifying Benefits, Impacts, and Needs.* Washington, D.C.: National Commission on Libraries and Information Science.

McCullough, Michael E., William T. Hoyt, David B. Larson, Harold G. Koenig, and Carl Thoresen. 2000. "Religious Involvement and Mortality: A Meta-Analytic Review." *Health Psychology* 19:211–22.

McGinnis, Kathleen, and James McGinnis. 1984. "Parenting for Peace and Justice." *Spirituality Today* 36:34–46.

McManus, Susan A. 1996. *Young v. Old.* Boulder, Colo.: Westview Press.

Mee, Cheryl L. 2003. "Geriatric Nursing." *Nursing* 33:8.

Memletics. 2004. "Adult Education, Employment and the Current Economic Climate." www.memletics.com/manual/adult-education.asp

Mentors Peer Services. 2004. "Mentor Services and Organizations that Specialize in Mentoring." www.peer.ca/mentorlinks.html

Mercury News. 2003. "Members of Church Claim Harassment." October 12. www.fva.org/2003 10/story08.htm

Metchnikoff, Elie. 1908. *The Prolongation of Life.* New York: G. P. Putnam's.

Meyrowitz, J. 1985. *No Sense of Place.* New York: Oxford University Press.

Mezey, Mathy, Christine Cassel, Melissa M. Bottrell, Kathryn Hyer, Judith Howe, and Terry T. Fulmer. 2002. *Ethical Patient Care: A Casebook for Geriatric Health Care Teams.* Baltimore: Johns Hopkins University Press.

Milbank Memorial Fund. 2000. *Pioneer Programs in Palliative Care.* Robert Wood Johnson Foundation.

Miller, Geri. 2003. *Incorporating Spirituality in Counseling and Psychotherapy.* New York: John Wiley & Sons.

Miller, Melvin, and Susanne R. Cook-Greuter. 2000. *Creativity, Spirituality, and Transcendence.* Stamford, Conn.: Ablex Publishing Corporation.

Miller, Michael B. 1979. *Current Issues in Clinical Geriatrics.* New York: Tiresias Press.

Millett, John. 2003. "Environmental News." www.epa.gov/agingrelease.pdf

Milner, Colin. 2002. "The Six Dimensions of Wellness for Older Adults." *Fitness Management* October: 56–59.

Minkler, Meredith, and Carroll Estes, eds. 1991. *Critical Perspectives on Aging.* Amityville, N.Y.: Baywood Press.

Mital, Parikh. 2003. "Networking Research." Morse.uml.edu/~mpirikh/research_mpirikh.html

Mitchell, Gail. 1999. "Empowering Caregivers." www.caregivers.com/pages/experts/goalsarticle.html

Mitchell, Olivia, ed. 1993. *As the Workforce Ages.* Ithaca: ILR Press.

Mitchell, Susan. 2001. *Generation X: Americans Aged 18 to 34.* Ithaca, N.Y.: New Strategist Publications.

———. 2003. *American Generations,* 4th ed. Ithaca, N.Y.: New Strategist Publications.

Moon, Marilyn. 2001. "Medicare Reform." Washington, D.C.: Urban Institute. www.urban.org/urlprint.cfm?ID=7327

Morano, Marc. 2003. "Networks Blamed for Using Political Activists as Repeat 'Victims'." July 14. http://www.cnsnews.com/ViewNation.asp?Page=%5 CNation%5Carchive%5C200307%5CNAT20030714a.html

Morgan, Carol M., and Doran J. Levy. 2002. *Marketing to the Mindset of Boomers and Their Elders.* St. Paul, Minn.: Attitudebase.

Morgan, Edmund S. 2002. *Benjamin Franklin.* New Haven, Conn.: Yale University Press.

Morrison, R. Sean. 2000. "Planning and Providing Care at the End of Life." www.hosppract.com/issues/2000/10/eldmoor.htm

Morrow-Howell, Nancy, James Hinterlong, and Michael Sherraden, eds. 2001. *Productive Aging.* Baltimore: Johns Hopkins University Press.

Moschis, George P. 1996. *Gerontographics.* New York: Quorum Books.

MoveOn.org. 2004. *Fifty Ways to Love Your Country.* Maui: Inner Ocean Publishing.

Moyle, Wendy. 2002. "Nursing Students' Perceptions of Older People." *Australian Journal of Nursing* 20:508–14.

Mullan, Phil. 2000. *The Imaginary Time Bomb*. London: I. B. Touris.

Muller, Robert. 2002. *Paradise Earth*. www.robertmuller.org

Mulligan, Casey B., and Xavier Sala-i-Martin. 1999. "Gerontocracy, Retirement, and Social Security." National Bureau of Economic Research Paper No. w7117.

Munshi, Sunil Kumar, Narayanaswamy Vijayakumar, Nicholas A. Taub, Harneeta Bhullar, T. C. Lo, and Graham Warwick. 2001. "Outcome of Renal Replacement Therapy in the Very Elderly." *Nephrology, Dialysis, Transplantation* 16:128–33.

Murray, Margo. 2001. *Beyond the Myths and Magic of Mentoring*. San Francisco: Jossey-Bass.

Myrdal, Gunner. 1944. *An American Dilemma*. New York: Harper.

Nader, Ralph. 2004. "What the Press Is Not Reporting." *Common Dreams Newscenter*. www.commondreams.org/views03/0822-07.htm

Nascher, I. L. 1914. *Geriatrics*. Philadelphia: P. Blakiston's Son and Co.

National Academy for Teaching and Learning about Aging. 1999. "What Do You Call Old People?" www.cps.unT.edu/natla/web/Call.html

National Academy of Science. 2004. "Project RISE." www.nas.edu/rise/examsel.htm

National Academy on an Aging Society. 1999. *Demography Is Not Destiny*. Washington, D.C.: Gerontological Society of America.

National Cancer Institute. 2004. "Spirituality in Cancer Care." www.nci.nih.gov/cancerinto/pdq/supportivecare/spirituality/healthprofessional

National Center for Education Statistics. 2002. *Participation Trends and Patterns in Adult Education, 1991 to 1999*. Washington, D.C.: U.S. Department of Education.

National Center for Health Statistics. 2003. *Health, United States. Special Excerpt: Trend Tables on 65 and Older Population*. Washington, D.C.: Government Printing Office.

National Conference of Catholic Bishops. 2001. "Environmental Justice: A Public Policy Framework." www.thegoodsteward.com/article.php3?articleID=364

National Council on the Aging. 1974. *Myths and Realities of Aging*. Washington, D.C.: NCOA.

National Grandparents Day. 2004. "About National Grandparents Day." www.grandparentsday.com/short_ver/htm

National Institutes of Health, National Institute on Aging. 1986. *Age Words: A Glossary on Health and Aging*. Bethesda, Md.: NIH.

National League for Nursing. 1988. *Strategies for Long-Term Care*. New York: National League for Nursing.

National Organization for Women. 2004. "The Promise Keepers." www.now.org/issues/right/06/04/pk.html

Nattier, Jan. 1997. "Buddhism Comes to Main Street." www.urbandharma.org/udharma/mainstreet.html

Naylor, Michele. 1999. "Adult Development." *PENpages*. www.penpages.psu.edu/penpages_reference/28507/285072634.HTML

Neighborhood Revitalization Strategies. 2002. Seattle's 2001–2004 Consolidated Plan, Appendix B.

Nelson, Douglas W. 1982. "Alternative Images of Old Age as Bases for Policy." In Bernice L. Neugarten, ed. *Age or Need?* Beverly Hills, Calif.: Sage Publications.

Nelson, Todd, ed. 2002. *Ageism.* Cambridge, Mass.: MIT Press.

Neuberger, Richard L., and Kelley Loe. 1936. *An Army of the Aged.* Caldwell, Id.: Caxton Printers.

Neugarten, Bernice L., and Robert J. Havighurst. 1976. *Social Policy, Social Ethics, and the Aging Society.* Washington, D.C.: Government Printing Office.

Neustadt, Richard E., and Ernest R. May. 1986. *Thinking in Time.* New York: Free Press.

New Democrats Online. 2004. "Idea of the Week: A Boomer Corps." www.ndol.org/ndol_ci.cfm?contentid=252331&kaid=131&subid=192

New York Times. 2004. "Pension Tension," editorial, August 8, *Week in Review,* 10.

Noonan, David, and Mary Carmichael. 2003. "A New Age for AARP." *Newsweek,* December 1.

Northcott, H. 1975. "Too Young, Too Old—Aging in the World of Television." *The Gerontologist* 15:184–86.

Novick, Peter. 1999. *The Holocaust in American Life.* Boston: Houghton Mifflin.

Nuland, Sherwin. 1994. *How We Die.* New York: Knopf.

Nunberg, Geoffrey. 2004. "Geezers, Gerries, and Golden Agers," *New York Times,* March 28, Week in Review, 7.

OASIS. 2003. "The Oasis Mission." www.oasisnet.org/about/index.htm

Oberlander, Jonathan, and Theodore R. Marmor. 2002. "The Pincher Strategy." *Campaign for America's Future.* www.ourfuture.org/projects/next_agenda.ch4_2.cfm

Office of Vocational and Adult Education (OVAE). 2004. "Adult Education Facts at a Glance." www.ed.gov/about/offices/list/ovae/pi/AdultEd/aefacts.html

Ohsako, Toshio. 1998. "Learning and Social Participation by Senior Citizens in Japan." UNESCO: Institute for Education.

Olshansky, S. Jay, and Bruce A. Carnes. 2001. *The Quest for Immortality.* New York: W. W. Norton.

Ore Module. 2004. "Different Age Groups." www.olc.org/ore/3age.htm

Orloff, Judith. 2001. "Health and Spirituality." www.shirleymaclaine.com/spirituality/healthspirit.html

Ottaway, Susannah, L. A. Botelho, and Katharine Kettredge, eds. 2002. *Power and Poverty.* Westport, Conn.: Greenwood Press.

Palmer, Parker. 1999. *The Active Life.* San Francisco: Jossey-Bass.

Palmore, Erdman. 1999. *Ageism.* New York: Springer Publishing.

Park Ridge Center. 2001. "Catholic Nun Explores Spirituality of Alcoholics Anonymous." May. www.parkridgecenter.org/Page1004.html

Parsons, Cynthia. 1999. *Mentors Strengthen Student Community Service.* Chester, Vt.: SerVermont.

Paul, Susanne. 1995. "Report from the Older Women's Tent at the NGO Forum in Beijing." *Aging International* 22:53–56.

Pavon Rabasco, Francisco Antonio, Ruiz Castellanos, and Inmaculada Ortiz Marquez. 2001. "An Educational Experience with Elderly People." www.uni-ulm.de/LiLL/prov2/europa/europaworkshop2001/beitraege/cadiz_en.html

Peacock, James R., Dana Burr Bradley, and Dena Shenk. 2001. "Incorporating Field Sites into Service-Learning as Collaborative Partners." *Educational Gerontology* 27:23–35.

Pear, Robert. 2003. "Sweeping Medicare Change Wins Approval in Congress; President Claims a Victory. *New York Times,* November 26, 1.

———. 2004. "AARP, Its Eye on Drug Cuts, Urges Changes in New Law." *New York Times,* January 17, A12.

Penn State. 1988. "Parent Aide Project." http://agexted.cas.psu.edu/dpcs/21600396.html

Persky, Trudy. 2004. "Overlooked and Underserved." *Mental Health and Aging.* www.mhaging.org/info/olus.html

Peterson, Peter. 1999. *Gray Dawn: How the Age Wave Will Transform America—and the World.* New York: Times Books.

Peterson, Peter, and Neil Howe. 1988. *On Borrowed Time.* San Francisco: ICS Press.

Petrella, Robert J. 1999. "Exercise with Older Patients with Chronic Disease." *Physician and Sportsmedicine* 27:1–12.

Pew. 2004. "Internet and American Life." www.pewinternet.org/reports/toc/asp?Report=106

Pew Forum on Religion and Public Life. 2003. "Religion and Politics." http://pewforum.org/docs/index.php?DocID=26

Phillipson, Chris. 1998. *Reconstructing Old Age.* London: Sage Publishing.

Pifer, Alan, and Lydia Bronte. 1986a. "The Aging Society." *Daedalus* 115 (Winter).

———. 1986b. *Our Aging Society.* New York: W. W. Norton.

Pillemer, Karl, and D. Finkelhor. 1988. "The Prevalence of Elder Abuse." *The Gerontologist* 28:51–57.

Pillemer, Karl, Phyllis Moen, Elaine Wethington, and Nina Glasgow, eds. 2000. *Social Integration in the Second Half of Life.* Baltimore: Johns Hopkins University Press.

Pitkin, Walter B. 1932. *Life Begins at Forty.* New York: McGraw-Hill.

Place, Michael D. 2000. "Health Coverage 2000." The Catholic Health Association of the United States. www.connective.com/events/health2000/agenda.html

Place, Nick T., Tracy Irani, and Chris Mott. 2003. "Adult Education in Extension." *Proceedings of the 19th Annual Conference.* Raleigh, N.C.: AIAEE.

Plain Language. 2004. "Writing User-Friendly Documents." www.blm.gov/nhp/NPR/pe_toc.html

Pleck, Elizabeth. 1991. "Childhood." In *The Reader's Companion to American History,* ed. Eric Foner and John A. Garraty. Boston: Houghton Mifflin.

Pope, Elizabeth. 2003. "Second Class Care." *AARP Bulletin Online.* November.

Porter, Debbie. 2004. "Chautauqua." www.nd.edu/~rbarger/www7/chautauqua
.html

Porter, Gareth, and Janet Welsh Brown. 1991. *Global Environmental Politics.*
Boulder, Colo.: Westview Press.

Posner, Richard. 1995. *Aging and Old Age.* Chicago: University of Chicago
Press.

Potter, Alicia. 1998. "As You Lay Dying." www.weeklywire.com/ww/archives/
authors/boston_aliciapotter.html

Praize. 2004. "Holy Apostles College and Seminary." www.praize.com/engine/
info/13192.html

Pratt, Henry J. 1976. *The Gray Lobby.* Chicago: University of Chicago Press.

———. 1993. *Gray Agendas.* Ann Arbor: University of Michigan Press.

Preservation Seattle. 2002. "July 2002: Chinatown International District."
www.cityofseattle.net/commnty/histsea/preservationseattle/neighborhoods/
defaultjuly.htm

President's Council on Bioethics. 2003. *Beyond Therapy: Biotechnology and the
Pursuit of Happiness.* October. http://bioethicsprint.bioethics.gov/report/
beyondtherapy/chapter4.html

President's New Freedom Commission on Mental Health. 2002. Meeting Min-
utes. www.mentalhealthcommission.gov/minutes/octo2.htm

President's Research Committee on Social Trends. 1933. *Recent Social Trends,*
2 vols. New York: McGraw-Hill.

Prevention. 1999. "Recruiting Older Volunteers for Prevention Programs."
www.health.org/govpubs/prevalert/v3i7.htm

Primedia. 2004. "Alcoholics Anonymous." http://atheism.about.com/library/
glossary/general/bldef_alcoholicsanonymous.htm

Proctor-Smith, Marjorie. 1995. *Praying with Our Eyes Open.* Nashville, Tenn.:
Abingdon Press.

Promise Keepers. 2004. "Ecumenical 'Macho-Men' for Christ?" www.rapidnet
.com/~jbeard/bdm/Psychology/pk/pk.htm

Putnam, Jackson K. 1970. *Old-Age Politics in California.* Stanford, Calif.: Stanford University Press.

Putnam, Robert D., and Lewis M. Feldstein. 2003. *Better Together.* New York:
Simon & Schuster.

Quality of Life Matters. 2002. "Hospice Care Linked to Superior Pain Management in Dying Nursing Home Patients," 1.

Qualls, Sara Honn, and Norman Abeles. 2000. *Psychology and the Aging Revolution.* Washington, D.C.: American Psychological Association.

Quill, Timothy E. 1989a. "Recognizing and Adjusting to Barriers in Doctor-
Patient Communication." *Annals of Internal Medicine* 111:51–57.

———. 1989b. "Utilization of Nasogastric Feeding Tubes in a Group of Chron-
ically Ill, Elderly Patients in a Community Hospital." *Archives of Internal
Medicine* 149:1937–41.

———. 1996. *A Midwife through the Dying Process.* Baltimore: Johns Hopkins
University Press.

Quintance, Alice. 2004. "Uncle Bob." www.realchangenews.org/pastarticles/
features/articles/fea.santos.html

Radiant Justice. 2000. "Recommendations of the Mayor's Justice 2000 Task Force, Grand Rapids, Michigan." http://radiantjustice.tripod.com

Radin, Eric L., and W. Andrew Achenbaum. Forthcoming. *Dysfunctional Doctoring.*

Ramalho Correia, Ana Maria. 2002. "Information Literacy for an Active and Effective Citizenship." www.nclis.gov/libinter/infolitconf&meet/papers/correia-fullpaper.pdf

Randall, Kate. 2003. "The Politics of US Medicare 'Reform': Cynicism, Cowardice, and Social Reaction." www.wsws.org/articles/2003/jun2003/medi-j30_pm.shtml

Rapoport, Nancy B., and Bala G. Dharan, eds. 2004. *Enron.* New York: Foundation Press.

Reddie, Anthony G. 2001. *Faith, Stories, and the Experience of Black Elders.* London: Jessica Kingsley Publishers.

Reed, C. C., S. C. Beall, and L. A. Baumhover. 1992. "Gerontological Education for Students in Nursing and Social Work." *Educational Gerontology* 18:625–36.

Reichel, William, ed. 1978. *The Geriatric Patient.* New York: HP Publishing.

Reilly, Sabrina. 2003. "NCOA Begins Civic Engagement Initiative." *Innovations* 2:10.

Rich, J. Scott, and Harold C. Sox. 2000. "Screening in the Elderly: Principles and Practice." *Hospital Practice.* www.hosppract.com/issues/2000/10/eldrich.htm

Riker, David. 1997. *U.S. Multinationals, and Competition from Low Wage Countries.* Cambridge, Mass.: National Bureau of Economic Research.

Riley, Matilda White, Robert L. Kahn, and Anne Foner, ed. 1994. *Age and Structural Lag.* New York: Wiley Interscience.

Riley, Matilda White, and John W. Riley. 1986. "Longevity and Social Structure." In *Our Aging Society,* ed. Alan Pifer and Lydia Bronte. New York: W. W. Norton.

Ritts, Vicki. 2000. "Culture and Aging." www.stlcc.edu/vritts/aging.html

Robinson, B. A. 2001. "Religious Practices in the U.S.: Poll Results." www.religioustolerance.org/chr_prac.htm

Robinson, Barrie. 1994. "Ageism." http://socrates.berkeley.edu/~aging/ModuleAgeism.html

Robinson, Thomas E., II. 1998. *Portraying Older People in Advertising.* New York: Garland Publishing.

Rogers, Anita. 1995. "Mentoring in Life Skills by Senior Citizens." www.nal.usda.gov/pavnet/ye/yelinkli.htm

Rohr, Richard. 1998. "Boys to Men." *Sojourners* 27 (May–June): 16–21. www.sojo.net

Rosenthal, Bruce. 2001. "Faith-Based Organizations Discuss Long-Term Care with HHS Secretary." www.aasha.org/public/press_release

Rother, John. 2004. "Why Haven't We Been More Successful Advocates for Elders?" *Generations* 28:55–58.

Rothkopf, David J. 2004. "Aging 'Haves' Pitted against Young 'Have-Nots'."

March 29. http://seattletimes.nwsource.com/text/2001889620_sundayclash28.html

Rotstein, Gary. 2003. "Health Officials Loath to Accept 'Old Age' as a Cause of Death." *Pittsburgh Post-Gazette.* www.post-gazette/pg/03257/221773.stm

Rozwenc, Edwin C., and Thomas Bender. 1978. *The Making of American Society,* 2 vols. New York: Alfred A. Knopf.

RUAH. 2004. "About Us." www.ruahspirit.org/about.html

Russell, Cheryl. 1999. *The Baby Boom: Americans Aged 35 to 54,* 2d ed. Ithaca, N.Y.: New Strategist Publications.

———. 2003. *Demographics of the U.S.: Trends and Projections,* 2d ed. Ithaca, N.Y.: New Strategist Publications.

RVY. 2000. "My Cancer Journal Essays: Year 1." www.phoenix5.org

Safford, Florence, and George I. Krell. 1992. *Gerontology for Health Professionals.* Washington, D.C.: National Association of Social Workers.

Saito, Rebecca N., and Eugene C. Roehlkepartain. 1992. "The Diversity of Mentoring." *Search Institute.* www.search-institute.org/archives/tdm.htm

Salvation Army. 2004. "Quick Facts about the International Salvation Army." www.salvationarmy-usaeast.org/world/army/index.shtml

Sanders, Arthur B. n.d. *Emergency Care of the Elder Person: Instructor's Manual.* New York: SAEM.

Sarton, May. 1973. *As We Are Now.* New York: W. W. Norton.

Schacter-Shalomi, Zalman. 2004. "Our Bodies, Ourselves." www.spiritualeldering.com

Schaie, K. Warner, and Carmi Schooler, eds. 1998. *Impact of Work on Older Adults.* New York: Springer Publishing.

Schick, Frank L., and Renee Schick, eds. 1994. *Statistical Handbook on Aging Americans.* Phoenix, Ariz.: Oryx Press.

Schleppegrell, Mary. 1987. "The Older Language Learner." *ERIC Digests.* www.ericdigests.org/pre-927/older.htm

Schneider, Margaret. 1937. *More Security for Old Age.* New York: Twentieth Century Fund.

Schull, Diantha. 2004. "Public Libraries: Places for Renewal." *Aging Today.* www.asaging.org/at/at-244/IF_Public_Libraries.cfm

Search Institute. 1995. "The Diversity of Mentoring." www.search_institute.org/archives/tdm.htm

Seattle Post-Intelligencer. 2004. "In Transition, But Still a Melting Pot." http://seattlepi.nwsource.com/webtowns/town.asp?WTID=6

SeniorCitizens.com. 2004. "Education." www.seniorcitizens.com/education/education.htm

Senior Corps. 2004a. "RSVP Program." www.seniorcorps.org/joining/rsvp

———. 2004b. "Foster Grandparents Programs." www.seniorcorps.org/joining/fgp

———. 2004c. "Senior Companion Program." www.seniorcorps.org/joining/scp

SeniorNet. 2004a. "About SeniorNet." www.seniornet.org

———. 2004b. "SeniorNet Learning Centers." www.seniornet/org

Sheldon, J. H. 1948. *The Social Medicine of Old Age*. London: Nuffield Foundation. Arno Reprint, 1980.

SHEM Center for Interfaith Spirituality. 2004. "Shem Programs." www.shemcenter.org/jobopenings.html

Shepherd, Jill. 1999. "Elderly Should Receive the Same Cancer Care as Young People." *British Medical Journal*. www.eurekalert.org/pub_releases/1999-07/BMJ-Esrt-300799.php

Shriner, Joyce A. 1996. "Rituals in Family Life." http://ohioline.osu.edu/flm97/curr.html

Simon, Jean Hurley. 2004. Testimony before U.S. Special Committee on Aging. http://aging.senate.gov/oas/f6js.htm

Simon, S., and J. Gurwitz. 2003. "Drug Therapy and the Elderly." *Clinical Pharmacology and Therapeutics* 73:387–93.

Simonton, Dean Keith. 1988. *Scientific Genius*. New York: Cambridge University Press.

Smith, James. 2004. "Anti-Aging Medicine." *Journal of Gerontology: Biological Sciences* 59a:649–709.

Smith, Ralph. 1979. *The Subtle Revolution*. Washington, D.C.: Urban Institute.

Solidarity. 2004. "Solidarity and Social Justice." www.justpeace.org/solid.htm

Solomon, Robert C. 2002. *Spirituality for the Skeptic*. New York: Oxford University Press.

Spickard, James V. 1995. "Body, Nature and Culture in Spiritual Healing." http://newton.uor.edu/FacultyFolder/Spickard/BodyNat.htm

Spicker, Stuart F., Stanley R. Ingman, and Ian R. Lawson. 1987. *Ethical Dimensions of Geriatric Care*. Boston: D. Reidel Publishing.

Spiritual Eldering Institute. 2004. "Volunteer Solutions." www.spiritualeldering.org

Spiritual Elders of Mother Earth. 2004. www.spiritualelders.org

Stanczak, Gregory C., and Donald E. Miller. 2002. *Engaged Spirituality*. University of Southern California: Center for Religious and Civic Culture.

Stanford, Eric. 2001. "Landmarks of Blessings." www.abc-usa/inmissn/summo1/summo1b.htm

Star-Gates. 2004. "An Alternative Healing Site." http://members.tripod.com/~medicinedreams/

State Initiatives. 2001. "How End-of-Life Care Can Be a Positive Issue for Policy Leaders." Issue 9:1–6.

St. Bartholomew's Episcopal Church, New York City. "The Center for Religious Inquiry." www.stbarts.org/cri.htm

Steere, David A. 1997. *Spiritual Presence in Psychotherapy*. New York: Bruner/Mazel.

Stern, Gary. 2003. "Mainline Protestants Reeling." *JournalNews.com*. May 4. www.nynews.com/newsroom/050403/a0104mainline.html

Stevens-Roseman, Ellen. 2004. "Working for a Living." *Journal of Jewish Communal Service* 80:169–74.

Stewart, Carlyle Fielding, III. 1999. *Black Spirituality and Black Consciousness*. Trenton, N.J.: Africa World Press.

Stolberg, Sheryl Gay, and Milt Freudenheim. 2003. "AARP Support Came as Group Grew 'Younger.'" *New York Times,* November 26, 1.

Stone, Robyn I., with Joshua M. Wiener. 2001. "Who Will Care for Us?" Report for the U.S. Department of Health and Human Services.

Strawbridge, W. J., R. D. Cohen, S. J. Shema, and G. A. Kaplan. 1997. "Frequent Attendance at Religious Services and Mortality over 28 Years." *American Journal of Public Health* 87:957–61.

Streim, Joel E. 2003. "Ageism in the Health Care System." Testimony before the Senate Special Committee on Aging, Washington, D.C.

Strom, Stephanie. 2003. "For Middle Class, Health Insurance Becomes a Luxury." *New York Times,* November 16, 25.

Stubblefield, Harold W. 1988. *Towards a History of Adult Education in America.* London: Croom Helm.

Suchman, Tony, Penny Williamson, John Cronin, and Diane Robbins. 2000. "Striking Moments in Relationship-Centered Care." www.fetzer.org

Sullivan, Kevin J. 2002. "Catching the Age Wave: Building Schools with Senior Citizens in Mind." Washington, D.C.: National Clearinghouse for Educational Facilities.

Swift, Jonathan. 1726. *Gulliver's Travels.* New York: Signet [1960].

Tallis, Raymond, and Howard M. Fillit. 2003. *Brocklehurst's Textbook of Geriatric Medicine and Gerontology,* 6th ed. Livingstone, U.K.: Churchill.

Thompson, Simon B. N. 1997. *Dementia.* Brookfield, Vt.: Ashgate Publishing Company.

Thompson, Warren S., and P. K. Whelpton. 1930. "A Nation of Elders in the Making." *American Mercury* 19:391–96.

———. 1933. "The Population of the Nation." In *Recent Social Trends: Report of the President's Research Committee on Social Trends.* New York: McGraw-Hill Book Co.

Thorndike, Edward L., Elsie O. Bergman, J. Warren Tilton, and Ella Woodyard. 1928. *Adult Learning.* New York: Macmillan.

Tirrito, Terry, and Toni Cascio, eds. 2003. *Religious Organizations in Community Services.* New York: Springer Publishing.

Tocqueville, Alexis de. 1836–1840a. *Democracy in America,* ed. Richard D. Heffner. New York: Mentor [1956].

———. 1836–1840b. *Democracy in America,* ed. J. P. Mayer. Garden City, N.Y.: Doubleday & Co. [1969].

———. 1836–1840c. *Democracy in America,* ed. Phillips Bradley. 2 vols. New York: Vintage Books [1945].

Toffler, Alvin. 1970. *Future Shock.* New York: Random House.

Toner, Robin. 2004. "Voters Are Very Settled, Intense, and Partisan, and It's Only July." *New York Times,* July 25, 1.

Tonks, Alison. 1999. "Medicine Must Change to Serve an Ageing Society." *British Medical Journal* 319:1450–51.

Torres-Gil, Fernando. 1992. *The New Aging.* Westport, Conn.: Auburn House.

———. 1999. "Aging and Latinization of California." *San Francisco Chronicle.* November 21. www.sfgate.com/cgi-bin/article.cgi?file=/chronicle/archive/1999/11/21/SC33888.DTL

Torres-Gil, Fernando, and TsuAnn Kuo. 1998. "Social Policy and the Politics of Hispanic Aging." *Journal of Gerontological Social Work* 30:143–58.

Tseng, Yueh-hsia, and Christine Mueller. 2001. "Elderly Volunteers and Service Credit Programs." *Research for Nursing Practice.* www.graduateresearch .com/Tseng.htm

Tuccillo, John, Buddy West, and Betsy West. 1995. *Targeting the Over 55 Client.* Dearborn Financial Publishing Co.: Real Estate Education Co.

Tunstall, Jeremy, ed. 1974. *The Open University Opens.* Amherst: University of Massachusetts Press.

Tupper, Meredith. 1995. "The Representation of Elderly Persons in Primetime Television Advertising." www.geocities.com/athens/8237/

Twentieth Century Fund Committee for Old Age Security. 1936. *The Townsend Crusade.* New York: Twentieth Century Fund.

United Nations. 2000. "Steps Towards a Society for All Ages." www.un.org/ esa/socdev/iyop/iyoppre3.htm

———. 2003. "Ageing." www.un.org/esa/socdev/ageing

University of Phoenix. 2002. "The Nation's Leading Online University." http:// online.phoenix.edu

U.S. Administration on Aging. 2004. "Elders and Families: Volunteer Opportunities." http://aoa.gov/eldfam/Volunteer_Opps/Volunteer_Opps.asp

USA Today. 2004. "Science Panel Urges Universal US Health Insurance by 2010." January 14. www.usatoday.com/news/health/2004-01-12-insurance panelx.htm

U.S. Bureau of the Census. 1960. *Historical Statistics of the United States, Colonial Times to 1957.* Washington, D.C.: Government Printing Office.

U.S. Conference of Catholic Bishops. 2003a. "Women's Spirituality in the Workplace." www.nccbuscc.org/laity/women/focusgroups.htm

———. 2003b. "Catholic Men's Ministries." www.nccbuscc.org/laity/marriage/ menministry.htm

U.S. Department of Health and Human Services. 2000. *Healthy People 2010,* 2 vols. Washington, D.C.: Government Printing Office.

U.S. Department of Labor, Bureau of Labor Statistics. 2004. *Volunteering in the United States, 2003.* Washington, D.C.: Government Printing Office.

U.S. Department of Labor, Women's Bureau. 2003. www.dol.gov/wb

U.S. Department of State. 2004. "Adult Education Opportunities." www.state .gov/m/dghr/flo

Usher, Robert, Ian Bryant, and Rennie Johnston. 1997. *Adult Education and the Postmodern Challenge.* London: Routledge.

U.S. Senate, Special Committee on Aging. 2003. "The Image of Aging in Media and Marketing." Serial no. 107-35. Washington, D.C.: Government Printing Office.

U.S. Senate, 108th Congress, 2nd Session, Committee on Health, Education, Labor, and Pensions. 2004. Resolution. www.grandparentsforchildren.org/ news.htm

Van Ryzin, Jean. 2004. "As Basic as ABC: Coalition Works to Bring Drug Savings to Lower-Income Medicare Beneficiaries." *Innovations* 33:6–9.

Van Tassel, David, and Jimmy Elaine Wilkinson Meyer, eds. 1992. *U.S. Aging Policy Interest Groups.* Westport, Conn.: Greenwood Press.

Vara, Richard. 2004. "Lawson to Retire from Wheeler Avenue Baptist." June 7. www.chron.com/archives

Vincent, John A. 1999. *Politics, Power and Old Age.* Buckingham, U.K.: Open University Press.

Visser, Roemer, and Paulette T. Beatty. 2003. "Managing an Aging Workforce." Bryan: Texas A&M University.

Wajnryb, Ruth. 2003. "When Old Euphemisms Pass Their Youth-by Date." www.smh.com.au/articles/2003/11/14/1068674365443.html

Waken, Daniel. 2003. "As Some Churches Falter and Others Grow, Catholic Church Plans Overhaul." *New York Times,* October 26.

Walker, David M. 2002. "U.S. Developing and Economic Trends and Related Developing World Implications." Speech to the National Academy of Social Insurance. October 31. www.gao.gov/cghome/demandecon/imgo.html

———. 2003. "Challenges and Opportunities of Aging Populations." Speech to AARP and the Woodrow Wilson Center. April 24. www.gao.gov/cghome/aging/index.html

Walker, Joanna, ed. 1996. *Changing Concepts of Retirement.* New York: Arena.

Walker, Rob. 2005. "Middle Age? Bring It On." *New York Times Magazine,* January 30, p. 30.

Wall, Steve. 1993. *Wisdom's Daughters: Conversations with Women Elders of Native America.* New York: HarperPerennial.

Walsh, Mary Williams. 2004a. "Voters Release Houston from Pension Law." *New York Times,* May 17, C2.

———. 2004b. "Bailout Feared If Airlines Shed Their Pensions." *New York Times,* August 1, A1.

———. 2004c. "Healthier and Wiser? Sure, but Not Wealthier." *New York Times,* June 13, C1.

Wasch, William K. 2004. "Establishment of the Susan B. and William K. Wasch Center for Retired Faculty." Wesleyan University press release.

Washington Post. 2003. "Right-to-Die Group Drops 'Hemlock' from Its Name." July 22. www.washingtonpost.com/ac2/wp-dyn?pagename=article&note=&content

Webb, Gisela. 1995. "Expressions of Islam in America." www.islamfortoday.com/america11.htm

Welford, A. T. 1958. *Ageing and Human Skill.* Oxford: Oxford University Press.

Wells Fargo Elder Services. 2004. "ASA Awards." Catalog, American Society on Aging/National Council on the Aging annual meeting, 328.

Werner, Carol. 2000. "Adult Education Philosophies: What's That Got to Do with Teaching Adults?" *TEAL Resources.* www.llcc.cc.il.us/TEAL/Philosophies.htm

Wiebe, Robert. 1967. *The Search for Order, 1877–1920.* New York: Hill and Wang.

Wilentz, Sean. 1984. *Chants Democratic.* New York: Oxford University Press.

Will, George (archive). 2002. "Europe." October 29. www/townhall.com/columnists/georgewill/gw20021029.shtml

Wills, Garry. 1994. *Certain Trumpets*. New York: Simon & Schuster.

Wilson, Kenneth G. 1993. "Senior Citizen." *The Columbia Guide to Standard American English* www.bartleby.com/68/80/5380.html

Wing Luke Asian Museum. 2004. "Seattle's Chinatown-International District." www.wingluke.org/international_district.html

Wolfe, David B., with Robert E. Snyder. 2003. *Ageless Marketing*. Dearborn, Mich.: Dearborn Trade Publishing.

Woolhandler, Steffie, and David U. Himmelstein. 2002a. "National Health Insurance: Liberal Benefit, Conservative Spending." *Common Dreams News Center*. www.commondreams.org/views02/0525-06.htm

———. 2002b. "Paying for National Health Insurance—And Not Getting It." *Health Affairs* 21:88–98.

Yadurajan, K. S. 2004. "Learn to Be Politically Correct with Words." www.deccanherald.com/deccamherald/mar252004/edu6.asp

Yang, Zhou, Edward C. Norton, and Sally C. Stearns. 2003. "Longevity and Health Care Expenditures: The Real Reasons Older People Spend More." *Journal of Gerontology: Social Sciences* 58B:S2–10.

Yntema, Sharon, ed. 1997. *Americans 55 and Older*. Ithaca, N.Y.: New Strategist Publications.

Yorks, Lyle, and Elizabeth Kasl. 2002. *Collaborative Inquiry as a Strategy for Adult Learning*. San Francisco: Jossey-Bass.

INDEX

AARP: changing image, 145; global aging initiative, 137; and health policy, 96–97, 144–145; and learning, 66; and older workers, 34, 39, 138; as policy advocates, 144, 145
Academy of Religion and Mental Health, 124
Adams, James Truslow, 56
adult education, 17–18, 51; 53–57; current trends, 61–65
advanced directives, 93
Adventist Development and Relief Agency, 108
advertisements, for/about aged, 41–44
Africa, population aging, 2
African Americans, 24, 41; community building, 110–111, 133, 148; demography, 6, 22; education, xiv, 17, 51–52; employment, 10–11; health and illness, 14–16, 90, 113, 155; spirituality, 106, 121
age: and employment, 8–10; and health, 13–16; and illness, 79–80, 85–86; and religion, 18–19
age and aging, 19, 60, 102, 160; in U.S. history, xiii–xv, 1
Age Discrimination in Employment Act, 31

ageism, 5, 27, 43, 93 160; defined, 78; in health care, 77–91, 102; link to racism, sexism, 91; in market, 31–32, 48; in media, 40–44
"Ageless Marketing," 46–48
AIDS, 114; in later years, 15, 89
alcohol, 14, 89; abuse, 125–126
Alcoholics Anonymous, 125
Alliance for Aging Research, 94–96
"alternative" late-life arrangements, 12; living, 23–24; work, 37–39
Alzheimer's disease, 14–15, 82
American Chemical Society, 73
American College of Physicians, 82
American Federation of Labor, 56
American Geriatrics Society, 78
American Medical Association, 82, 154
American Pharmaceutical Association, 154
American Psychological Association, 124
Americans for Generational Equity, xviii, 136–137
American Society of Internal Medicine, 82
American Society on Aging, 120
andragogy, 58–59
anti-aging medicine, 2

New Age mysticism, 125
Newman, Sally, 69
9/11 and unilateralism, 135
Nixon, Richard, 141
Nuland, Sherwin, 93
nursing, geriatric, 83
nursing homes, 22, 80, 107; composition of, 16, 90, 96; problems in
91–92

OASIS, 66–67
obesity, 115
occupational patterns, 7–8, 27–28
old age, adaptability in, 126; disease or decay, 77, 80; meaning transformed, 159–160
old-age dependency, xiv
older Americans: as activists, 107, 128, 144; as burdens or contributors, 126, 128, 155; as consumers, 44–48; as older learners, 59–60; as patients, 79, 82–83, 90, 95–96, 101; and religion and spirituality, 106, 108, 114, 116, 119, 122–123; as social capital, 66; term, objectionable, 130
Older Americans Act, 34
older workers, current options, 30, 37–39; diversity of, 39; images of, 8, 27, 31, 39; and Social Security, 36;
old-fogyism, 50; research undercuts, 57
"old-old," 91; demography of, 5, 21, 39, 117; health of, 15–16, 80–81, 86
On Lok Senior Health, 96, 147
Open University, U.K., 62
Osler, William, 76–77
osteopaths, 81

palliative care, 153
part-time employment, 11–12, 37–38
Patient Self-Determination Act, 154
Peace Corps, 70
pediatrics, 83
Pension Benefit Guaranty Corporation, 144
Pentecostalism, 105; among Hispanics, 106
Pepper, Claude, 146
Peterson, Peter, xix
Pfizer, 47

philanthropies, 56, 55; fund more to youth than age, 71–72
Pifer, Alan, xvii
political behavior of older Americans, 19–21; civic engagement, 131, 146–148; contrast with young, 20–21; at federal level, 143–145; neoconservative, 141–143; political initiatives, abroad, 139–140
population aging: alarm over, xviii–xix, 136–137, 159; demography of, xi, 2, 99, 136, 186; and global aging, 135–136; interest in, xvi–xix, 97; need for productive elders, 23–24, 131
prayer, 104, 113, 121; efficacy of, 111
Presbyterian Church, 105
Prescription Drug Improvement and Modernization Act, 98, 144–145
preventive medicine, 80, 85–86; elderly ignored in, 88–89
private insurance companies, 102
productivity, 24; elders as source of, 160; Japanese initiatives, 138–139
Program on Age & Structural Change, xviii
Programs of All-Inclusive Care for the Elderly (PACE), 96
prolongation of life, 2–3
Promise Keepers, 123–124
psychoneuroimmunology, 112

Quill, Timothy, 155
Quinlan, Karen Ann, 94

race: and employment, xiv, 11; differences in health, 13, 15–16
racism, 91
radio and older learners, 56
Ramalho Correira, Ana Maria, 131
religiosity: and health, 93, 112–114; pluralistic, 104–107; and spirituality, 128; varies, 110
religious beliefs and practices: age-based, 18, 19; attendance and affiliation, 104–106; about dying, 153, 155; and well-being, 115–116
respite care, 152
Retired and Senior Volunteer Program (RSVP), 67, 69

About the Author

W. Andrew Achenbaum received his Ph.D. in history from the University of Michigan. A professor of social work and history at the University of Houston, he heads the Gerson David Consortium on Vital Aging. He has also taught at Canisius College, at Carnegie Mellon University, and, for most of his career, at the University of Michigan, where he was a professor of history and deputy director of its Institute of Gerontology.

Achenbaum is the author of five books and co-editor of eleven others. His first book, *Old Age in the New Land* (Johns Hopkins, 1978), was selected by *Choice* as an academic book of the year. A past board chair of the National Council on the Aging, Achenbaum has also been a delegate to two White House Conferences on Aging and served on the advisory board of the Carnegie Corporation's Aging Society Project.